VALUES-BASED DECISION-MAKING FOR THE CARING PROFESSIONS

David Seedhouse

Auckland University of Technology, New Zealand
and Middlesex University, London, UK

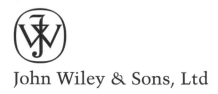

John Wiley & Sons, Ltd

Other Wiley Editorial Offices

John Wiley & Sons Inc., 111 River Street, Hoboken, NJ 07030, USA

Jossey-Bass, 989 Market Street, San Francisco, CA 94103-1741, USA

Wiley-VCH Verlag GmbH, Boschstr. 12, D-69469 Weinheim, Germany

John Wiley & Sons Australia Ltd, 33 Park Road, Milton, Queensland 4064, Australia

John Wiley & Sons (Asia) Pte Ltd, 2 Clementi Loop #02-01, Jin Xing Distripark, Singapore 129809

John Wiley & Sons Canada Ltd, 22 Worcester Road, Etobicoke, Ontario, Canada M9W 1L1

Wiley also publishes its books in a variety of electronic formats. Some content that appears in print may
not be available in electronic books.

Library of Congress Cataloging in Publication Data

Seedhouse, David, 1956–
  Values-based decision-making for the caring professions / David Seedhouse.
     p.   cm.
  Includes bibliographical references and index.
  ISBN 0-470-84734-4 (alk. paper) — ISBN 0-470-84735-2 (pbk : alk. paper)
  1. Medical personnel—Decision making.   2. Medical care—Decision making.   3. Values.   I. Title.

  R723.5.S44 2005
  362.1'068'3—dc22

                                                                        2005044308

British Library Cataloguing in Publication Data

A catalogue record for this book is available from the British Library

ISBN-13 978-0-470-84734-3 (HB) 978-0-470-84735-0 (PB)
ISBN-10 0-470-84734-4 (HB) 0-470-84735-2 (PB)

Typeset in 10/12pt Palatino by Integra Software Services Pvt. Ltd, Pondicherry, India
Printed and bound in Great Britain by Antony Rowe Ltd, Chippenham, Wiltshire
This book is printed on acid-free paper responsibly manufactured from sustainable forestry in which
at least two trees are planted for each one used for paper production.

For those who care enough to think about their values

Contents

About the Author

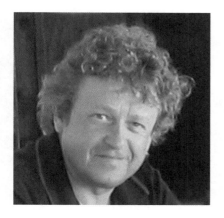

David Seedhouse is a truly original thinker and prolific author, highly regarded by health practitioners, teachers and students alike. Though David has a background in philosophy, his work is always focussed on solving practical problems.

Professor Seedhouse is best known for his writing on health and ethics, yet his work straddles many areas of social, philosophical and political concern. He has written or edited 14 books and produced over 200 book chapters, journal papers and other articles. His library includes the highly successful editions of *Health: The Foundations for Achievement* and *Ethics: The Heart of Healthcare*; the full list of his titles is given at the back of this book.

His primary interest now lies in the development of software to enable transparent decision-making in health care, local democracy, schools and other social settings. The considerable practical impact of David's work can be seen – and engaged with – at www.values-exchange.com.

David is Professor of Health and Social Ethics at Auckland University of Technology, New Zealand (where he directs the National Centre for Health and Social Ethics) and Professsor of Health Care Analysis at Middlesex University, London. He is CEO of VIDe Ltd – www.vide.co.nz – and a popular keynote conference speaker internationally.

Preface

We are not machines, yet we allow society to programme us to do what reason dictates, mostly without any struggle at all.

From pre-school to the grave, we meekly conform to rational ways of life that are plainly not in our interests. We take test after test because schoolteachers tell us to, we lock adult rule-breakers away in cruel and crowded prisons, we medicate our children when life excites them, and we adhere slavishly to military protocols as we exact revenge on foreign infidels. If anyone challenges these absurdities, the first reaction is to wave the rule book at them, and if that doesn't work to beat them until they see the light. Rarely if ever do we regard our fellow human beings as catalysts for growth. We would much rather they did as they were told than try to understand their unique experience of life – and so we miss opportunity after opportunity to grow.

I have a hero whose desire to think for himself has always been an inspiration to me. Philosopher and iconoclast, Paul Feyerabend thought more deeply and more broadly than I can, but I think I am in some ways pursuing the same project. When he died, Feyerabend was writing a book called *Conquest of Abundance*,[1] which was published posthumously. In it he shows how we abstract a mere handful of features from life's astonishing richness, and foolishly enshrine them as SCIENTIFIC REALITY or THE TRUE WAY TO LIVE.

> In trying to see the wood all the time, we have lost sight of the trees. The wood may be the correct image for SOME problems, but the individual trees are also the correct image for other problems. And no procedure exists to tell us beforehand what the correct image may be.[2]

Values-Based Decision-Making is offered in this spirit. It explains why we need comprehensive decision transparency, and describes the beginnings of an ambitious project to achieve it. This practical venture uses software which enables its users to express their feelings and arguments by means of common concepts, and feeds back structured reports which can compare their perceptions with thousands of other people's.

Perhaps this process might itself be conceived as a diminution of abundance: directing people's minds towards particular questions and organising their responses into categories is bound to distract from alternative insights at some point. However, the project is exceedingly ambitious. We are building an international values exchange (values-exchange.com), able to reveal an exhilarating depth of feeling, thinking and practical possibility for every imaginable subject. The **Values Exchange**® not only enhances our understanding of different points of view, it fosters deeper and deeper communication between people who would never otherwise encounter each other.

At the moment (2005) the **Values Exchange** is used primarily to explore health care situations and options, but its methods and subjects are already evolving. Ultimately, the Values Exchange will promote:

> ...the freedom of human beings to confront the richness of being and extract meaning from it with tools that themselves change their meaning as they are used.[2]

To see our logical and emotional selves in proper proportion, to seek otherness and difference, continually to use intellect and imagination to ask: 'what if....?', to embrace our human nature without trepidation. This, I like to think, is what Paul Feyerabend had in mind.

David Seedhouse
Torbay, Auckland, New Zealand
May 2005

Acknowledgements

I would like to thank Craig Evans, Ben Liebert, Mike Clist, and Technology New Zealand for helping me build the software described in this book. I would also like to thank Auckland University of Technology for tolerating my determination to go my own way; and Hilary, Charlotte and Penny (my family) for being the most perfect 'work distractions' I could ever hope for.

Introduction

More and more we find existential comfort in our technical achievements. We communicate at lightening speed, we have sovereignty over our genes, we gaze at atoms through computerised microscopes, and we have formulae designed to overcome all manner of illness and anguish.

Our technology is so pervasive, and we think so much of it, that we are losing sight of what we really are – biological, emotional, evaluative beings, desperate for meaning.

We acknowledge our sensitive qualities, but only as a backcloth to our lives. Mostly we are content to leave them to those on the margins of technology – to poets, playwrights, artists and dreamers. Or worse, we see our sensitivities as problems. We caution ourselves to distrust our intuitions, to shun value judgements, to resist the emotional response. Time after time we resolve to decide rationally, in accord with the evidence – and nothing but the evidence.

It's as if we've erased the clause:

THE POST-HOLDER IS REQUIRED TO BE FULLY HUMAN

from our job descriptions. We are becoming super-technicians – high on protocol, down on passion – like the emotionally disconnected surgeon I stumbled into a few years ago.

WHAT GOOD IS A BLUNT SURGEON?

On the third day of the Test Match I felt my mouth fill with blood. I was already anxious and miserable because I was to have a tumour removed the next Tuesday. But finding the blood shattered me. I had no idea what to do. I was in a crowd, but I spat the blood out in a panic until it stopped (which it did after a few minutes). I found out – after frantic phone calls to various doctors – that it was a 'side-effect' of a needle biopsy done two days earlier, and 'nothing to worry about'.

The surgeon who performed the biopsy had not only neglected to explain what he was going to do before he took the sample from my lump, but had also failed to inform me of any of the five adverse consequences that might result (one of which, I later discovered, was a gush of blood in the mouth).

Surely a classic example of bad ethics and woeful communication, and a horrible experience that I could have been spared. And now, as I reflect on what happened (with the operation behind me), I think it was worse than this. I think I encountered pure farce.

I discovered this in bed, recovering from the operation. I was watching a comedy film – a poor imitation of a Sellars burlesque in which the Sellars sound-alike was playing a crack-pot General. A piece of dialogue went something like this:

Soldier: Sir, Sir. The enemy are storming our lines. What shall we do?
General: Shoot the soldiers you idiot.
Soldier: What about the tanks, Sir?
General: Do they have soldiers in?
Soldier: (*Exasperated*) How do I know? What difference does it make?
General: I'm infantry my man. My job's shooting soldiers. Best to leave the hi-tech stuff to the boffins, what?

Not exactly a side-splitting interchange, but it stuck in my memory because the General was plainly my surgeon. The General's basic problem was not his nuttiness, but the lack of a Master Plan. His job was to kill soldiers, anything beyond that was not his concern.

My surgeon thinks his job is to be technically efficient, to follow the surgical text-book to the letter. Anything more – reflection on the broader inspiration for his calling, for instance – is not his business.

A damaging parody of the crackpot General, my surgeon works to relieve patients of physical pain and disease – and so of the concomitant anxiety these problems cause – but he sees no point in trying to reduce other fears by explaining causes and consequences. He did not even think it important to tell me the result of the biopsy.

My surgeon would not be pleased, I imagine, if his anaesthetist were to control only muscular pain and ignore neuralgia, yet he saw nothing ironic in helping physically while doing nothing to enable me to cope with my associated problems, worries typically experienced by anyone who discovers a tumour.

Of course not every surgeon behaves so insensitively, but many do. And they do so largely because we spend millions teaching medical students to be good technicians and still – decades after the principle has apparently been accepted by medical educators – we devote a mere pittance to the human side of medicine.

It is just laughable that for all the humane declarations of pompous medical leaders, medical schools to this day award professional degrees to students proficient with medical technology yet brainless about the point of using it.[3]

In most organisations, whenever a decision needs to be made the call is for 'evidence', 'clear-headedness', 'objectivity', 'reason' – for some way of deciding what to do independent of the people who have to make the decision. The last thing organisations seem to want is human feeling, which is typically regarded as too biased, too vague or too ephemeral to be depended on.

Unquestionably, evidence and reason are essential to good decision-making. Without them we are ignorant and foolish. But why do we rate evidence and reason so much higher than our emotional powers? Why do we consider our human preferences of so little consequence? What have we got against values?

'NOTHING BUT' LOGIC

Herbert A. Simon, a twentieth-century computer scientist, famously compared *Homo sapiens* to the ant:

> An ant, viewed as a behaving system, is quite simple. The apparent complexity of its behaviour over time is largely a reflection of the complexity of the environment in which it finds itself... At the level of cells or molecules, ants are demonstrably complex; but these microscopic details of the inner environment may be largely irrelevant to the ant's behaviour in relation to the outer environment. That is why an automaton, though completely different at the microscopic level, might nevertheless simulate the ant's gross behaviour...
>
> I should like to explore this hypothesis, but with the world 'man' substituted for 'ant'...
>
> A man, viewed as a behaving system, is quite simple. The apparent complexity of his behaviour over time is largely a reflection of the complexity of the environment in which he finds himself... I myself believe that the hypothesis holds even for the whole man.[4]

According to Simon, the inner environment of the 'whole man' (sic) – his biology, his thoughts, his beliefs, his poetry – is 'largely irrelevant' to what he does. Whole man merely responds to problems thrown at him by the environment he inhabits.

Simon is convinced that all human responses can be copied by machines:

> I have surveyed some of the evidence from a range of human performances, particularly those that have been studied in the psychological laboratory.
>
> The behaviour of human subjects in solving cryptarithmetic problems, in attaining concepts, in memorizing, in holding information in short-term memory, in processing visual stimuli, and in performing tasks that use natural languages provides strong support for these theses... They are simple things, just as our hypothesis (that the inner environment of the whole man is irrelevant to his behaviour) led us to expect. Moreover, though the picture will continue to be enlarged and clarified, we should not expect it to become essentially more complex. Only human pride argues that the apparent intricacies of our path stem from a quite different source than [sic] the intricacy of the ant's path.[5]

In other words human beings are little more than stimulus-response organisms, with an embarrassingly inflated view of our intellectual and emotional importance. If we are hungry, we will find food. If we are threatened we will fight or try to escape. If one set of information is more important to our survival than another, we will privilege it in our short-term memory store. Just like ants.

It is easy to claim that people are machines. But just because our behaviours are largely predictable and depend on our circumstances, this does not mean there is nothing interesting or important going on behind the behavioural scene. While it is true that:

> ...the behaviour of human subjects in solving cryptarithmetic problems, in attaining concepts, in memorizing, in holding information in short-term memory...[5]

mostly uses logic (and can be copied and in many cases greatly improved upon by computer programmes) we also have other, quite different responses. Our reactions to the plight of others, to moral problems, to the demands of ageing, to spiritual crises, to political choices and countless other social challenges reveal and require a different dimension of human existence.

Simon is a super-technician *par excellence*. His view of human life stems from his scientific approach. Like the rest of us, scientists are attracted to phenomena they can easily interpret and manipulate. Understandably, they tend to disregard those things that respond less readily to their methods. Joseph Weizenbaum explains that:

> Science can proceed only by simplifying reality. The first step in its process of simplification is abstraction. And abstraction means leaving out of account all those empirical data which do not fit the particular conceptual framework within which science at the moment happens to be working...[6]

Weizenbaum likens this to the well-known joke in which a policeman comes across a drunk, on his knees, searching for something under a lamppost. He tells the officer he lost his keys 'over there', pointing into the darkness. 'In that case why are you looking for them over here?' the policeman asks. The drunk replies, 'Because the light is so much better here'.

Weizenbaum quotes Aldous Huxley:

> Pragmatically [scientists] are justified in acting in this odd and extremely arbitrary way; for by concentrating exclusively on the measurable aspects of such elements of experience as can be explained in terms of a causal system they have been able to achieve a great and ever increasing control over the energies of nature. But power is not the same thing as insight and, as a representation of reality, the scientific picture of the world is inadequate for the simple reason that science does not even profess to deal with experience as a whole, but only with certain aspects of it in certain contexts. All this is quite clearly understood by the more philosophically minded men of science. But unfortunately some scientists, many technicians and most consumers of gadgets have lacked the time and the inclination to examine the philosophical foundations and background of the sciences. Consequently they tend to accept the world picture implicit in the theories of science as a complete and exhaustive account of reality; they tend to regard those aspects of experience which scientists leave out of account, because they are incompetent to deal with them, as being somehow less real than the aspects which science has arbitrarily chosen to abstract from out of the infinitely rich totality of given facts.[7]

Even more pointedly:

> Because of the prestige of science as a source of power, and because of the general neglect of philosophy, the popular Weltanschauung of our times contains a large element of what may be called 'nothing-but' thinking. Human beings, it is more or less tacitly assumed, are nothing but bodies, animals, even machines... values are nothing but illusions that have somehow got themselves mixed up with our experience of the world; mental happenings are nothing but epiphenomena... spirituality is nothing but... and so on.[8]

But values are not illusions. Not only are values and mental experiences very obviously real to everyone, they ARE us just as much if not more than our reason.

WE ARE SPONTANEOUS BEINGS

If I hear my child cry I can reason about it:

- I hear my child crying
- I decide her yelling sounds more like a cry for attention than a frightened cry
- I decide I shall therefore ignore her crying for the moment

If I hear my child cry I will also feel about it. Quite out of my logical control I will experience a range of sensations. Perhaps:

- Anxiety
- Love
- Cold
- An impulse to run
- Annoyance
- Guilt
- A heightened focus on sound
- Relief

It would seem very strange for any parent to say that feelings such as these are somehow less significant than logical analysis about what to do. The two aspects are intimately related – reason and experience can be used to moderate an emotional reaction, and emotions can override reason if a need is sensed. But they are quite plainly not automatically ranked:

1. **Reason (Dominant/Primary)**
2. **Emotion (Minor/Secondary)**

Why then, in business, health care, government and virtually any other non-religious human organisation, do we pretend that our spontaneous nature is less important or less real than our reason?

Of course, practical concerns tend to dominate when you are trying to cure disease or make money. Tried and trusted rules and procedures develop over time – laws, protocols, decision-trees, probability analyses – and it often makes good sense to use them. But it doesn't always make sense. Problems for which there are no neat protocols, or where the rules are open to interpretation, arise continually (see **Chapter 4**, p. 103 and **Chapter 5** p. 121, for example). And immediately they do we begin to flounder. Since we have turned our backs on our evaluative nature, what else can we expect?

The most common consequence of our floundering is that we confuse technical expertise with expertise in values. We call upon technical experts not only to decide issues within their field of competence; we also ask them to make judgements about the USE of that field, as if the two aspects are obviously related. Mental health tribunals, for example, require psychiatrists to determine what risk a patient will be if discharged. Yet psychiatrists are trained in medicine, not risk-assessment or value judgement.

Technical proficiency and expertise in values are no more related than know-how in soccer is related to advising on the desirability of wage caps for soccer players; or expertise in growing vegetables is related to skill in landscape gardening. There may be a relationship, but more than likely there won't be. And almost always there will be non-technicians better placed to offer the required advice, since they will be much less inclined to mistake their (lack of) technical knowledge for moral authority.

ARE WE AFRAID OF OUR VALUES?

I believe we have exaggerated the reach of technical rationality because we distrust and even fear our values. There's something wild and uncontrollable about them. And these days we super-technicians are used to being in charge. So we spurn our values and as a result lock away the largest part of our nature.

But we are wrong to worship evidence and technology the way we do. And we shouldn't be afraid. As soon as you understand what a value is you can see that while people may have unequal access to evidence, and unequal technical ability to assess it, everyone (even children) has exactly the same access to our values, and exactly the same ability to apply them in our decision-making.

WHAT IS A VALUE?

It is very easy to understand what a value is. It would be possible to write a scholarly treatise on the subject (one or two academics have already done so), but it is not really necessary. There are potential intricacies, as there are with any human concept, but there is little practical value in pursuing them.

A handful of writers appreciate that values are central to human affairs. For example, Milton Rokeach writes:

> It is difficult for me to conceive of any problem social scientists might be interested in that would not deeply implicate human values.[9]

And G.W. Allport says:

> A value is a belief upon which a man acts by preference.[10]

Rokeach offers these rather bookish definitions:

> A *value* is an enduring belief that a specific mode of conduct or end-state of existence is personally or socially preferable to an opposite or converse mode of conduct or end-state of existence. A *value system* is an enduring organisation of beliefs concerning preferable modes of conduct or end-states of existence along a continuum of relative importance.[11]

Rokeach, Allport and I take a similar view of values. If we were to debate the point, we might possibly disagree about whether values must be acted upon to be values (I don't think it's necessary, though Allport does). However, we all agree that values come about as a result of human preferences: no preferences, no values.

In an academic arena I might also take issue with Rokeach's five assumptions about the nature of human values, which are:

> 1) The total number of values that a person possesses is relatively small; 2) all men every-where possess the same values to different degrees; 3) values are organised into values systems; 4) the antecedents of human values can be traced to culture, society and its institutions and personality; 5) the consequences of human values will be manifest in virtually all phenomena that social scientists might consider worth investigating.[11]

I agree with assumptions 4 and 5. With regard to 4, where else other than our psychology, biology and social conditioning could our values possibly come from? And 5 is self-evident. However, in my view the only limit on how many values one can hold is the number of preferences one can hold – and we all hold very many preferences, consistent and inconsistent, all the time. But this is a trivial issue, depending merely on the meaning of 'relatively' in the quote above.

A little more importantly, unless I completely misunderstand Rokeach, it is not the case (2) that all men (sic) possess 'the same values to different degrees'. If:

> A *value* is an enduring belief that a specific mode of conduct or end-state of existence is personally or socially preferable to an opposite or converse mode of conduct or end-state of existence...[11]

as Rokeach claims, and if different people have conflicting preferences, then logically it cannot be the case that 'all men possess the same values', unless one sets up a very generalised conception of 'values'.

For example, if Bill has an enduring belief that daily exercise is personally preferable to no daily exercise while Gena takes the exact opposite view, then they must have different values. The only way they can have the same value is to say 'both Bill and Gena value physical well-being but seek it in different ways'. But if one says this then Rokeach's definition is undermined, since the general statement is not 'a specific mode of conduct', and we are left merely with a platitudinous set of values: we all value happiness, we all value health, we all value social cohesion and so on.

In fact a value does not need to be enduring to be a value – if I sincerely believe today that exercise is good for me then I value exercise – today the idea 'exercise is good' (at least for me) is one of my values. If I change my mind tomorrow then one of my values has changed for some reason. Simple as that.

With regard to Rokeach's 3), values can be arranged in values systems, or can be interpreted as being in values systems, but this doesn't mean they are actually and permanently set up in consistent hierarchies. They may be, for some people, but for most people there is flexibility and the possibility of change.

To illustrate, one can imagine a values system something like this.

Say a person has ten major values. From these, three might be selected as being especially relevant to conversations with work colleagues:

- Telling the truth
- Not inflicting avoidable pain on another person
- Protecting my own interests

These could be defined as a values system since for many situations they work coherently, for example, when establishing an equitable work rota. However, if a work colleague is not pulling her weight and this is impacting on you personally, the values need to be ranked to help decide whether or not you should report her to your boss. If you rank them:

1. Telling the truth
2. Not inflicting avoidable pain on another person
3. Protecting my own interests

you may decide merely to confront the slack employee, on the ground that 2 is more valuable than 3. However, if you rank them:

1. Telling the truth
2. Protecting my own interests
3. Not inflicting avoidable pain on another person

you may decide it is better for you to go straight to the boss.

Which ranking you decide upon is not implicit within these three values themselves, but will depend on another value (perhaps 'working in a successful business' or 'friendly relationships with as many colleagues as possible'). This deciding value may come from within the system or not – but there has to be some deciding value.

It is tempting to think we all have some unmoving, fundamental values which underpin everything we do. Robert Veatch, for example, came up with the expression 'deep values'. Veatch thinks the best chance of making accurate guesses about which treatment is in a patient's best interests is to pair patients with 'providers who share their deep values'. This would mean:

> ...picking providers on the basis of their religious and political affiliations, philosophical and social inclinations, and other deeply penetrating worldviews.[12]

However, because:

> (t)he value choices that go into a judgment about what is best for another are so complex and subtle...[12]

Veatch recognises that even clinicians who are paired for 'deep values' might not get the judgement right.

They wouldn't get it right because so-called deep values are themselves complex, variable and subject to change. I like to think I value equality and take a strong stand against discrimination between human beings. But while this is true in a general way, the fact is that I am prepared to compete with other people in order to win benefits for myself, and I am very selective about the people I spend time with and have as my students. What's more, my apparently less grand but much more visible values – my valuing gardening, swimming and drinking in bars – make no contribution whatsoever to my alleged deep values.

The truth is that although individuals do have sets of values that roughly define us, our values systems tend to be malleable dependent upon context – sometimes one value wins out, sometimes another, and not necessarily in any coherent or consistent way – simply because we are variable, emotional, biological creatures in social and personal flux.

To sum up, values are expressions of preference. Sometimes they are organised logically, sometimes they are not. Sometimes they are permanent, sometimes they are not. This variation matters little – it is an inevitability of life. What matters is that we see and understand our values for what they are.

WHAT IS A VALUE?

- In order for a human being to value some thing or process she must like it in some way
- Generally speaking, the degree to which a thing or a process is valued depends on the degree to which a person likes that thing or process, and this can vary between contexts and over time
- If a person has no preference toward a thing or a process she cannot be said to value it. If she dislikes a thing or a process in some way then she disvalues it, or values it negatively
- A value-judgement is a decision based upon a person's liking or disliking a thing or process
- All value-judgements stem from human feelings: 'I like this', 'I am drawn toward this', 'This makes me feel sick', 'I am afraid of this', 'I find this beautiful'
- Value judgements will almost always include evidence – good value judges take account of as much relevant evidence as they can
- A thing or a process can be valued absolutely (in its own right) or relatively (in comparison with other things or processes).

In sum:

A value is a human preference for a thing, a state, or a process

A value-judgement is a decision based upon one or more values

PART ONE

Mr Spock's Mistake

CHAPTER ONE

The Limits of Reason

SUMMARY

- Mr. Spock* advises us to deal firmly with our emotions and to rely on logic alone
- Despite its practical power, Spock-reason is never enough. Every time we examine it in context we soon run up against its limits. What at first seems sensible can quickly turn silly
- There are examples everywhere of the limits of evidence-based assessments and technical rationality. A mammography example is illustrative
- It is impossible for human beings to act in value-free ways – evidence and values are forever entwined in the social world
- For millennia we have wanted to split reason and passion. Yet this split is artificial and potentially destructive since it feeds the belief that human decisions can be made with the supposedly reasonable side of the split alone

$$\blacklozenge$$

The fictional Mr. Spock championed the use of logic over emotion, which he blamed for warfare and other violence. Half-Earthling, half-Vulcan, Spock argued that if humanity wants to live in peace we must learn to be less emotional. Ideally, we should do away with our emotions altogether.

According to *Star Trek* legend,[13] Vulcans have practised fastidious logical concentration for centuries. Beginning at the earliest possible age, Vulcan children are taught not to show emotion, even though they experience it:

> What you do not yet understand is that Vulcans do not *lack* emotion. This is an all too common misconception. It is merely that our emotions are controlled, kept in check. This adherence to principles of logic offers a serenity that humans rarely experience in full. We have emotions. But we deal firmly with them and do not let them control us. (Elder Spock to Young Spock in *Yesteryear*)[14]

The Vulcan ideal has an immediate and simple appeal. If logic is independent of emotion, then every logical problem-solver is bound to arrive at the same solution to the same

---

* The title of this part of the book is a deliberate parody of *Descartes' Error*, the title of a book by Antonio Damasio.

Values-Based Decision-Making for the Caring Professions   David Seedhouse
© 2005 John Wiley & Sons, Ltd

problem as any other logical problem-solver, guaranteeing consistent policy-making and social harmony.

Unsurprisingly, it turns out that things are not quite as simple as this.

SPOCK-REASON: SENSIBLE, SUSPECT OR SILLY?

Wherever there is a human problem you can be sure that someone somewhere is trying to find a Spock-rational strategy to solve it. In science, computing, mathematics, medicine, education, politics – even in theology and philosophy – an industry of people toils to find simpler, more elegant and less costly answers.[15–22]

All this effort to solve problems algorithmically* is not only often a good thing, it is inevitable. All species are driven to solve problems, and in our case the use of Spock-reason is obviously the best way to find many of the answers we need.

But what exactly is Spock-reason (or technical rationality)? More important, at what point does technical rationality stop and something else begin?

Undoubtedly, many uses of technical rationality are completely sensible. To try to solve problems any other way would be daft. But not all its applications are like this. There is a sliding scale:

1. **Sensible** – the best way to solve the problem at hand
2. **Suspect** – Spock-reason works, but leads to questionable or counter-intuitive results
3. **Silly** – to use Spock-reason alone to solve the problem is ludicrous.

SENSIBLE SPOCK-REASON

The classic assumptions of technical rational decision-making are that:

1. Problem-solvers seek or ought to seek maximum personal advantage on every occasion
2. Any problem can be extracted from the muddy flow of human life, separated from other problems, and dealt with as an exercise in logic.

Utility theory, for example, assumes that for any decision there must be an ordering by preference of all possible outcomes. These outcomes are given on a numerical scale which typically ranges from 0 to 1 or from 1 to 100, where the smallest number expresses the least desirable outcome and the highest represents the most preferred outcome (this ordering is said to create a 'utility function').[23] In conditions of uncertainty (i.e. pretty much always) utility theory says that people behave, or should behave, as if seeking to 'maximise their utility function'.

So far, so obvious. If I am in a situation in which my utility function indicates 89 for a strawberry ice cream, 87 for a coffee flavoured ice cream and 81 for a Popsicle, and I have enough money for only one choice, if I am Spock-rational I will choose the strawberry ice cream.

This simple example makes sense because deciding which flavour ice cream to buy given a fixed sum of money is a problem framed by assumptions 1 and 2 above (go for the tastiest and ignore everything else you might be doing).

---

* An algorithm is a precise rule – or set of rules – which specify how to solve a problem. The term typically refers to a recursive computational procedure for solving a problem in a finite number of steps.

This form of technical rationality also assumes that every alternative choice is known (i.e. there is no luscious pineapple split hiding at the bottom of the fridge), and the consequences of choosing each alternative can be fully ascertained (I will definitely enjoy the strawberry ice cream best). Traditional utility theory also assumes that decision-makers' desires can be ordered on a single scale, so that any two bundles of options can always be compared (apples with apples, pears with pears, ice creams with ice creams) and ranked so that when A is preferred to B, and B is preferred to C, then A is preferred to C.

DECISION TREE ANALYSIS – CHOOSING BETWEEN OPTIONS BY PROJECTING LIKELY OUTCOMES

Decision trees are a good example of the sensible application of technical rationality. They help their users decide what's best from several courses of action, using a logical structure and a clear picture of the risks and rewards associated with each possible option.

In order to create a decision tree the user must have multifaceted alternatives to choose from. The basic choice might be represented as a box at the left of a large piece of paper (**Figure 1**). Lines can be drawn from this box to represent each possible solution, the nature of which may be written along the line.

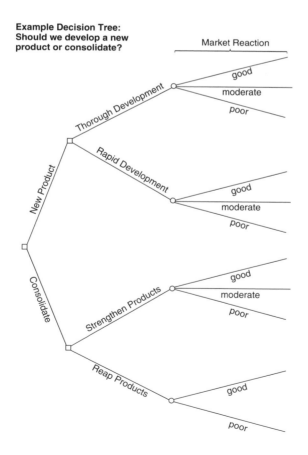

Figure I

The probable results of each solution can be noted at the end of each line. If the result is uncertain, a small circle can be drawn. If the result is another decision that needs to be made, another square can be drawn. The process can carry on until the user has drawn out as many of the possible outcomes and decisions as she can anticipate.

The tree diagram can be used for reflection and to stimulate further thought about possible solutions or outcomes not yet considered.[24]

Evaluating the decision tree

In order to work out which option has the greatest worth it is necessary to assign a cash value or a score to each possible outcome. It is also necessary to look at each circle and estimate the probability of each outcome. If historical data are available, rigorous estimates of probability may be possible.

This gives a tree like the one shown in **Figure 2**.

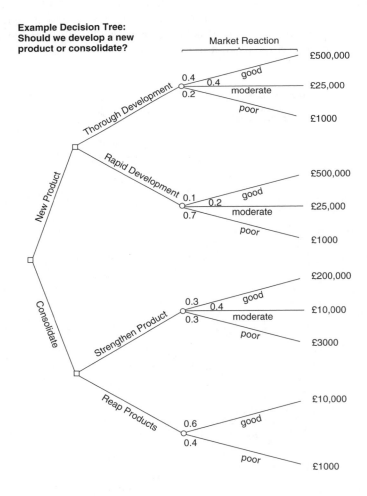

**Example Decision Tree:
Should we develop a new
product or consolidate?**

Figure 2

Calculating tree values

Once the value and probability of the outcomes has been decided, calculation is possible. The idea is to start on the right-hand side of the decision tree, and work back towards the left, recording calculations as they are made.

Calculating the value of uncertain outcome nodes

In order to calculate the value of uncertain outcomes (circles on the diagram) the value of the outcomes must be multiplied by their probability. The total for that node of the tree is the total of these values.

In the example in **Figure 2**, the value for 'new product, thorough development' is:

0.4 (probability good outcome)×£500,000 (value)=£200,000
0.4 (probability moderate outcome)×£25,000 (value)=£10,000
0.2 (probability poor outcome)×£1000 (value)=£200
Total=£210,200

Figure 3 shows the full calculation of uncertain outcome nodes. The values calculated for each node are shown in the boxes.

Calculating the value of decision nodes

In order to evaluate a decision node, the cost of each option must be written along each decision line, and then subtracted from the cost of the outcome value, in order to give a value that represents the benefit of that decision.

Once these decision benefits have been calculated, the rational choice is the option which gives the largest benefit.

Figure 4 shows the calculation of decision nodes in the example given.

In the example of **Figure 4**, the benefit for 'new product, thorough development' is £210,200. The future cost of this approach is estimated at £75,000, giving a net benefit of £135,200.

The net benefit of 'new product, rapid development' is £15,700. Therefore on this branch the option to choose is 'new product, thorough development', and in turn this alternative wins out over the option to consolidate.

Though obviously limited, decision trees provide an effective method of making some kinds of decision because they:

- Clearly lay out the problem so that all options can be reviewed and assessed
- Allow analysis of the possible consequences of decisions
- Provide a framework to quantify the values of outcomes and the probabilities of achieving them
- Help bring existing information and best guesses systematically to bear on decision-making

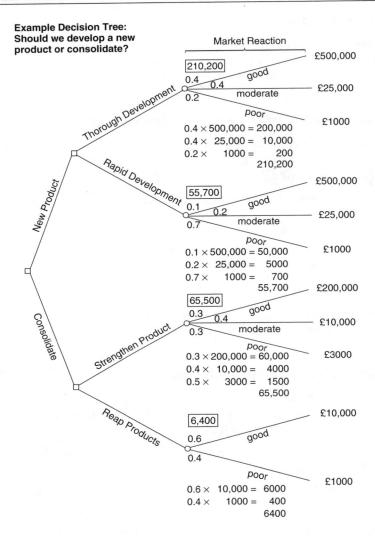

**Example Decision Tree:
Should we develop a new
product or consolidate?**

Market Reaction

Thorough Development

210,200
0.4   0.4   good   £500,000
0.2   moderate   £25,000
poor
0.4 × 500,000 = 200,000   £1000
0.4 × 25,000 = 10,000
0.2 × 1000 = 200
210,200

Rapid Development

55,700
0.1   0.2   good   £500,000
0.7   moderate   £25,000
poor
0.1 × 500,000 = 50,000   £1000
0.2 × 25,000 = 5000
0.7 × 1000 = 700
55,700

New Product

Strengthen Product

65,500
0.3   0.4   good   £200,000
0.3   moderate   £10,000
poor
0.3 × 200,000 = 60,000   £3000
0.4 × 10,000 = 4000
0.5 × 3000 = 1500
65,500

Consolidate

Reap Products

6,400
0.6   good   £10,000
0.4
poor   £1000
0.6 × 10,000 = 6000
0.4 × 1000 = 400
6400

Figure 3

If you have a small range of choices – if for example you are a start-up business with few products and you need to grow to stay competitive – then logical analysis of this sort unquestionably makes sense. But if things are more complex – say you are in a well-established business with many products and many choices about what to do with your profits – you are more likely to draw on a rather more mysterious method, on the edge of logic: 'business-instinct', 'common-sense' or perhaps 'intuition' ('it just feels right'), no matter how many decision trees you draw, and no matter how complex they are.

The edge of logic

You can see both the sense and the edge of logic by visiting http: // www.pointwizard.com/. *Point*Wizard* is a clever algorithm for computing an overall preference based on comparisons of different combinations of pairs. Without the algorithm, even for

**Example Decision Tree:
Should we develop a new
product or consolidate?**

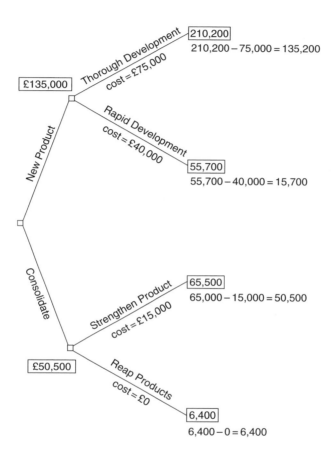

Figure 4

everyday decisions, there are millions of paired choices to sift through. *Point*Wizard*
typically reduces these to fewer than 50 decisions for most applications.

Possible uses of *Point*Wizard* include:

- managing hospital waiting lists
- appraising investment projects
- short-listing job applicants
- selecting immigrants
- admitting students to restricted courses
- identifying new product ideas for commercialisation
- choosing the best site for a building
- choosing which model of car to buy

Unlike the decision tree method, *Point*Wizard* has most value in situations where statistical
approaches, such as regression or conjoint analysis, are inappropriate or impossible.

Point*Wizard lets the decision-maker determine the relative importance of relevant criteria herself. The system analyses these subjective judgements to compute the most preferred decision choice.

Figure 5 is an example of the use of *Point*Wizard* in hiring staff. In this example there are 5 criteria with 2, 3 or 4 categories each. Instead of 'guessing' the relative importance of the criteria – their weights or scores – *Point*Wizard* allows the user to determine them in a methodical, transparent and repeatable way.

After the user has specified her criteria, *Point*Wizard* asks her to choose between 2 alternatives, where each is described according to 2 criteria at a time (**Figure 6**). The same type of choice is repeated using different alternatives until enough information about the user's preferences has been collected. In the hiring example, about 20 answers would be required.

After the user has answered the questions, *Point*Wizard* scores each alternative and ranks them automatically. It also creates a points system (**Figure 7**) that may be used to rank alternatives that may be unknown to the user.

a	Highest educational qualification
1	No qualifications
2	School-leaving certificate
3	Batchelors degree
4	Masters/doctorate

b	Amount of experience
1	<1 year
2	1 to 5 years
3	>5 years

c	Energy and enthusiasm
1	Poor
2	Good

d	Social skills
1	Not personable
2	Personable

e	Quality of references
1	Poor
2	Average
3	Good

Figure 5   (Misspelling of 'Bachelors' in original)

Which applicant would you prefer to hire?

a Highest qualification
    Bachelors
		a Highest qualification
		    PhD

c Years of experience
    3 to 10
	or	c Years of experience
		    Less than 3

This one		This one

They are equal

Figure 6

Name	Criteria					Score	Rank
	Highest educational qualification	Amount of experience	Social skills	Quality of references	Energy and enthusiasm		
Legolas Greenleaf	Masters/doctorate	>5 years	Personable	Poor	Poor	44	1
Sam Gamgee	Batchelors degree	>5 years	Not personable	Average	Good	35	2
Arwen	Batchelors degree	<1 year	Personable	Poor	Good	32	3
Bilbo Baggins	No qualifications	1 to 5 years	Personable	Good	Poor	30	4
Pippin Took	Masters/doctorate	1 to 5 years	Not personable	Good	Poor	29	5
Frodo Baggins	Masters/doctorate	>5 years	Not personable	Poor	Poor	28	6
Merry Brandybuck	No qualifications	<1 year	Personable	Average	Good	25	7
Gandalf the Grey	No qualifications	1 to 5 years	Personable	Poor	Poor	21	8
Galadriel	Batchelors degree	<1 year	Not personable	Average	Poor	19	9
Arogom	School-leaving certificate	<1 year	Not personable	Poor	Good	13	10

Figure 7   (Misspelling of 'Bachelors' in original)

Point*Wizard is certainly logical, but it does not produce Spock-rational answers in the sense that:

> . . . every logical problem-solver is bound to arrive at the same solution to the same problem as any other logical problem-solver . . . (p. 3 this text)

When using the system for ranking waiting lists for medical operations based on forms such as the example in **Figure 8**, the New Zealand Ministry of Health (a *Point*Wizard* customer) found that most doctors who make choices according to the method in **Figure 6** produce different results from the 'ideal' ranking. Even in the most apparently straightforward cases, upwards of 20 per cent of clinicians make decidedly 'wrong' choices, and hardly anyone gets a result exactly in line with the result he 'should' get.[25] Some of these 'inaccuracies' were caused by the Ministry's choice of criteria, which did not include age and more global understandings of quality of life for example, and some can be attributed to doctors 'clicking the wrong button'; nevertheless it seems that most clinicians prefer their own judgements to the official variety. The *Point*Wizard* system can accommodate additional criteria – like cost, confidence in the success of the operation and 'clinical judgement' (more of which later on) – so demonstrating how important it is to apply values comprehensively to apparently technical areas of decision making, and suggesting that we come close to the edge of logic surprisingly quickly.

Demo points system for orthopaedic surgery

Natural History of the potential or actual problem	Points	Score
Unlikely to deteriorate	0.0%	
May deteriorate or result in increased disability	5.0%	
Will probably result in increasing disability	5.5%	
Likely to progress to major complication or disability	12.9%	
Life or limb threatening	33.1%	

Pain

No pain	0.0%	
Intermittent activity related +/– analgesics	0.5%	
Episodic pain or incident related, but may be severe	1.2%	
Persistent pain with activity and at rest, regular analgesic, no sleep disturbance	6.7%	
Dominates life and regularly interferes with sleep	33.1%	

Personal functional limitation

Some difficulty but no limitation to personal activities	0.0%	
Moderate restriction to personal activities, e.g. requires intermittent help with some activities	3.1%	
Severe restriction to personal activities, e.g. requires daily help with dressing, toilet, shower	3.6%	

Social Limitation

Mild restriction, e.g. can walk up to an hour, unable to participate in sport	0.0%	
Moderate restriction, e.g. inability to work, can shop independently, can walk for up to half hour	6.9%	
Severe restriction, e.g. confined to property, requires help with shopping, can walk up to 10 minute	10.0%	

Potential to benefit from operation

No improvement likely	0.0%	
Small improvement likely	5.2%	
Moderate improvement likely	10.0%	
Substantial improvement likely	13.1%	
Return to near normal likely	20.2%	

Total score:

Figure 8

SUSPECT SPOCK-REASON

We can see from the *Point*Wizard* example that if technical rationality's calculations are to be plausible, they must somehow reflect the complexity and unpredictability of the real world. And yet Spock-reason cannot even begin to operate unless it makes major assumptions about the nature and stability of problems and problem-solving: most significantly, as we have seen, it must assume that problem-solvers are self-interested and that it makes sense for them to attempt to solve the problems they've chosen to solve, rather than any other problems they might be addressing.

SOME ELEMENTARY RULES FOR SPOCK-REASON

According to Spock-reason people are supposed to think consistently and system-atically, using concepts like these:

Dominance: A choice is said to be dominant if, when compared to another, it yields a superior outcome. For example, a car A is dominant to B if it is equal in all respects except that it provides more miles per gallon

Cancellation: If two risky alternatives include identical and equally improbable outcomes among their possible consequences, then the utility of these outcomes should be ignored in choosing between the two options. In other words, the choice should be made only on the basis of outcomes that differ

Continuity: For any set of outcomes, utility theory holds that a gambler should always prefer a gamble between the best and worst outcome to a sure bet inter-mediate position, if the odds of the best outcome are good enough. For example, a gambler should certainly prefer a gamble between £100 and complete financial ruin over a sure outcome of £10 provided the odds of financial ruin are, say:

$$1 \text{ in } 1,000,000,000,000,000,000,000,000,000,000,000,000$$

Invariance: If the mathematical outcomes are identical, a decision-maker should not be influenced by the way the alternatives are presented

TROUBLE IS, PEOPLE DON'T SEEM TO BE RATIONAL IN THE WAY WE'RE SUPPOSED TO BE

Naturally enough, study after study shows that these assumptions, and Spock-reason's many other rules, are repeatedly violated: most of the time people don't 'maximise their utility functions' or think in logical decision trees because people are, well…people. Indeed, the study of actual strategies used by major corporations to make their investments shows massive departures from Spock-reason (even though such corporations are presumably better-placed than anyone else to undertake scrupulously rational assessments).[26]

THE PRISONER'S DILEMMA

Anyone can experience this 'theory/reality' gap by attempting the Prisoner's Dilemma game. Its inventor, Albert Tucker, came up with this story:[27]

> Two burglars, Tony and George, are captured near the scene of a burglary. They are given the 'third degree' separately by the police. Each has to choose whether or not to confess and implicate the other. If neither man confesses, both will serve one year on a charge of carrying a concealed weapon. If each confesses and implicates the other, both will go to prison for 10 years. However, if one burglar confesses and implicates the other, and the other burglar does not confess, the one who has collaborated with the police will go free, while the other burglar will go to prison for 20 years on the maximum charge.

What is the most rational strategy in this situation? Arguably, Spock-reason requires both men to reason like this:

> My partner can confess or keep quiet. If he confesses and implicates me I'll get 20 years if I don't confess, 10 years if I do, so in that case it's best to confess. On the other hand, if he doesn't confess, and I don't either, I get a year, so in this case it's better not to confess. And yet, if I confess I can go free. So overall I stand the chance of most advantage if I confess. So I'll confess.

But if they both reason like this they both go to prison for 10 years. Whereas if they act counter to Spock-reason and keep quiet, they could escape with one year each.

The fact that individually rational action results in both burglars undermining their self-interest has had a wide impact in social science. Much real behaviour mirrors the Prisoner's

Dilemma: including arms races which create huge and useless stockpiles of weapons; the convenience of driving to work which leads to very inconvenient road congestion and pollution; and overfishing which causes depleted or even vanished fisheries.[28-30] In each case, rational action meant to maximise self-interest leads to results which ultimately damage it.

The subject has generated prolific academic debate and there are now all manner of different versions of the prisoner's dilemma game, including forms where rewards rather than punishments can be had. In these games players are able to make repeated decisions and so learn how the other player or players behave. In laboratory experiments with these forms of the game it is often found that players adopt a 'tit for tat' strategy: each is trustful or cooperative so long as the other is too. If one partner exploits the other on a particular trial, the other player implements the manipulative strategy on the next trial and continues to do so until the partner switches back to the trustful strategy. Under these conditions the game tends to stabilise – players continue to pursue the mutually trustful (though not utility maximising) strategy.[31]

To cope with the fact that people seem less Spock-rational than they should be, technical rationality's advocates invented a notion called subjective expected utility (**SEU**). Not unreasonably, **SEU** advises researchers to find out how an individual thinks of a problem as a human subject before judging whether she is rational or not.[32]

Within **SEU** there is a school of thought that assumes less than 'fully rational' choice.[33] For example, 'limited rationality' market theories presuppose that managers are aiming at 'satisfactory profits', or that their concern is to maintain market share, rather than to maximise profit, as they strictly should as wholly self-interested agents. 'Limited rationality theory' still takes for granted that economic agents want to maximise their utility, but within risky real world limits of incomplete information and uncertainty of outcome. Theories of this sort accommodate empirical evidence that people don't always seek to maximise utility (if we did no one would enrol in Christmas savings plans which offer interest at much less than the market rate).

Other formulations have been proposed to deal with the difference between ideal and real behaviour, the most well-known of which is called Prospect Theory.[34] Its inventors, Kahneman and Tversky, became interested in anomalies in risk-taking behaviour. They noticed that when people are offered a choice formulated one way they may be risk-averse, and yet when offered essentially the same choice in a different way they may display risk-seeking behaviour. For example, when given a choice between certainly getting $1000 or having a 50% chance of $2500 and a 50% chance of nothing, the researchers found that many people tend to choose the certain $1000 even though the mathematical expectation of the uncertain option is $1250. Conversely, the same people facing a certain loss of $1000 versus a 50% chance of no loss and a 50% chance of a $2500 loss will often eschew the certain loss in favour of the riskier alternative.

All this goes to show that however much you bend a rule of Spock-reason to cope with what we actually do, sooner or later a different human behaviour will force you to bend another one.

SILLY SPOCK-REASON

This said, there is clearly some sense in technical rationality. Equally clearly however, there are cliff-like limits to Spock-reason, and it doesn't take very long to run into them.

THE HEDONIC CALCULUS

Jeremy Bentham came up with a method of working out the sum total of pleasure and pain produced by an act. He called it the Hedonic Calculus (after hedone, the Greek word for pleasure), or the Felicific Calculus.[35] When determining what action is right in any given situation, Bentham advised that we should consider the pleasures and pains that might result from it, with regard to their *intensity, duration, certainty, propinquity* (closeness), *fecundity* (the chance that a pleasure will be followed by other pleasures, a pain by further pains), *purity* (the chance that pleasure will be followed by pains and vice versa), and *extent* (the number of persons affected). We should then consider alternative courses of action, comparing them according to the Calculus, until we can't think of any more. This process will reveal which act will produce the greatest balance of pleasure over pain and is therefore (according to Bentham) morally right. Bentham envisaged that his Calculus might be used for criminal law reform, ensuring that only the minimum punishment necessary for prevention would be handed out for a particular crime.[36]

Certainly there is something sensible about this, but there is much more about it that is just silly. For example, here is an extract from a paper called *Mathematics for Ethics*:[37]

> Ethical reasoning requires the consideration of values. If we represent the values numerically, we can use standard mathematical operations to manipulate them, and hopefully produce an answer which we can use to guide our actions...
>
> The initial problem is one of representation – how can we represent things like pain and pleasure with numbers? Presumably ... by using a scale. There are standard scales for distance (e.g. metres, kilometres, and miles etc.) and temperatures... There are no standard scales for pleasure and pain (that I know of) so we have to invent our own. The important thing is that we use the scale consistently, and that we make sure it is **linear** and **absolute**. I may not know exactly how far a mile is, but, because the mile scale is absolute, I know that 0 miles is no distance at all; and because it is also linear, I can be certain that one mile is exactly half the distance of two miles. Because we invent the scale, we can set it as we wish – to suit our particular problem – and it works fine so long as we use it consistently ...[37]

Well, no. It doesn't actually. We have a very good idea what a mile is because it is a conventional standard. Anyone can attempt to measure a mile and be right or wrong. Pain, on the other hand, is a subjective experience. No one else can measure my pain because no one else has access to it. This essential subjectivity means it is impossible to say objectively even that something is or isn't a pain (a sensation one person thinks of as painful may be pleasurable to another). Half a mile is half a mile. What half a pain is, is pretty much anyone's guess.

This ought to be enough to stop the *Mathematics for Ethics* project in its tracks. Yet it goes on undeterred:

> If we have a scale such that pleasures have a positive numerical value, then we can choose to represent pain and suffering on the same scale using negative numbers. For example, if I had a blister on my foot, I might think the pleasure from eating a chocolate

bar isn't worth the suffering it would take to walk to the shop and buy one – in which case, I can say the value of the suffering caused by me walking on a blistered foot is . . . more negative than –1.[37]

One might say such a thing, I suppose. However, one is much more likely to ask some-one else to bring the chocolate in, take a drive to the shop, eat something else instead (without worrying about all those empty calories), read a book, watch television, or burst the damn blister. Indeed, one is much more likely and well advised to do any of these things rather than take the hedonic or felicific calculus seriously:

> . . . whether or not it is worth limping to the shops depends on how long it will take me to get there . . . We can model this mathematically using multiplication: total suffering = average suffering per unit time * amount of time . . . by using the average suffering per unit time, I have not committed myself to the assumption that the suffering is constant – I may well find that suffering per unit time of walking on a blistered foot depends on how much walking I've already done on it. I can calculate the average amount of suffering per unit time over a given period of time using: average suffering per unit time = (suffering per unit time at the beginning of the period + suffering per unit time at the end of the period) / 2 as long as we assume a constant rate of change in the period.[37]

Why anyone would want to do this math becomes progressively more mysterious as the calculations grow in complexity:

> The situation [a different one from the case of the blistered foot – DS] is modelled by this tree:

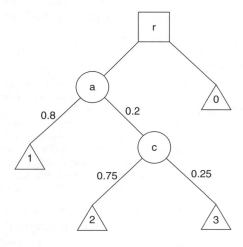

This gives the payoff values

- Node "0": 0
- Node "1": 1
- Node "2": $1 + (-2) = -1$
- Node "3": $1 + (-0.2) = 0.8$

We can now calculate the tree value, and from this learn which "branch" I should pick: I could, in a larger analysis, have many other branches (links) from the root node, indicating things I could choose to do *instead* of the particular act that I'm thinking of. I would then choose the node with the highest value. . . .

In this example, the expected value of "c" is:
(the probability of reaching node "2" * the value of node "2") + (the probability of reaching node "3" * the value of node "3")
$= (0.75 * -1) + (0.25 * 0.8)$
$= -0.75 + 0.2$
$= -0.55$

The expected value of "a" can now be calculated as:
(the probability of reaching node "1" * the value of node "1") + (the probability of reaching node "c" * the value of node "c")
$= (0.8 * 1) + (0.2 * -0.55)$
$= 0.8 + (-0.11)$
$= 0.69$

The next node up being a decision node, its value is simply the largest of node "a" and node "0":
$\max(0.69, 0) = 0.69$.

Since the expected value for node "a" is higher than that for node "0", and "a" represents what happens when I do this action, the tree therefore indicates that I *should* do the action (in preference to not doing it). If I could create a tree for a different course of action which (when using the same scale) returns a value greater than 0.69, then obviously I ought to do that instead.[37]

Obviously? In fact things have become very silly indeed – a corruption rather than simplification of reality.[1] Obviously any sensible person will choose the option which produces the greatest 'final quantitative utility value' for them (**Figure 9**). But just like other abstractions – like 'I'll act for the best' or 'I'm always fair' – it leaves the important questions unasked: why analyse this situation and not an alternative one? What happens when the unexpected occurs, as it inevitably will? What is the value (or disvalue?) of undertaking laborious mathematics when you have ten choices, or fifteen, or twenty-five? Right now I can go for a walk, a swim, go to the pub, keep on writing this, write a play, write a column, sit in the sun, go dig the garden, make a snack, stroke the cat, feed the goldfish, play with my children, paint the house, build a dog kennel, write a letter to the local newspaper, take a shower, have a nap … umpteen possibilities that only a lunatic would seriously bother to address with Spock-reason.

YOU CAN HAVE TOO MUCH OF A GOOD THING

Spock-reason gets silly so quickly because its advocates are obsessed with squeezing as much as they possibly can into their formulae, regardless of whether it makes any sense to do so. In the world outside Spock-reason, pretty much anyone can see it is nothing less than pathological to believe mathematics can tell you what to do ethically. It is a form of psychological denial: it denies that values are essential for every human decision; it denies that valuing is an emotional process, and it denies that we human beings NEED to value.

Spock-reason acknowledges emotions and values only because it has to: to get a utility function you have to have preferences. Once noted these preferences are placed to one side and ignored. It is almost as if emotions and values are an embarrassing little secret (um, yes, we all do it but we don't really need to talk about it, do we?).

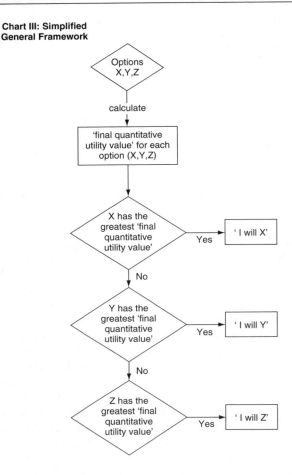

Chart III: Simplified General Framework

Figure 9[38]

While calculation is obviously part of good decision-making, the emphasis on the solely logical aspects has distorted our understanding of both how we make decisions and how we SHOULD make decisions. The technicalities have obscured the sources – and therefore the most important aspects – of decision-making.

Even Herbert. A. Simon is aware that there is more to decision-making than we normally associate with rationality:

> The very first steps in the problem-solving process are the least understood. What brings (and should bring) problems to the head of the agenda? And when a problem is identified, how can it be represented in a way that facilitates its solution? . . . While some problems are receiving full attention, others are neglected. Where new problems come thick and fast, 'fire fighting' replaces planning and deliberation. . . . relatively little has been accomplished toward analysing or designing effective agenda-setting systems . . .
>
> The way in which problems are represented has much to do with the quality of the eventual solutions . . . very different social welfare policies are likely to be proposed in response to the problem of providing incentives for economic independence than are proposed in response to taking care of the needy . . . the representation or framing of problems is even

less well understood than agenda setting. Today's expert systems make use of problem representations that already exist. But major advances in human knowledge derive from new ways of thinking about problems...[33]

The following example illustrates how important it is that we are clear about 'what brings problems to the head of the agenda'.

THE MAMMOGRAPHY DEBATE

In 1997 in the USA there was heated controversy about breast-screening for women aged forty years or more.[39] A National Institutes of Health (**NIH**) Consensus Conference came to the conclusion that:

> ...the data currently available do not warrant a universal recommendation for mammography for all women in their forties. Each woman should decide for herself whether to undergo mammography. Her decision may be based not only on an objective analysis of the scientific evidence and consideration of her individual medical history, but also on how she perceives and weighs each potential risk and benefit, the values she places on each, and how she deals with uncertainty.[40]

The Conference based its decision on its preferred interpretation of the available evidence,[41] namely:

- Routine screening of 10,000 women aged 40 to 49 will lengthen the lives of approximately 0 to 10 of them
- To lengthen one life, approximately 2500 women will have to undergo regular screening
- It is not known how long life will be prolonged for each woman
- Benefits from undergoing mammographic screening are more likely for women in their late 40s

The Conference warned that:

- A false-negative mammogram will almost certainly delay diagnosis and treatment
- A false-positive mammogram will prompt further testing, ordinarily by two of several possible invasive diagnostic methods
- Mammography is likely to cause anxiety, fear, and inconvenience. It could even decrease women's willingness to undergo screening mammography in later years, when the probability of benefit from the procedure is highest
- Some cancers grow so slowly that early detection is not crucial. Screening mammography may reveal such cancers and thus adversely affect insurance coverage
- Regular screening mammography will cause an increase in the diagnosis of ductal carcinoma in situ (DCIS), a category of noninvasive lesions that may or may not become invasive. Thus, there is a risk of overtreatment
- There is a hypothetical risk of breast cancer from mammographic radiation[42]

US Congress and the *New York Times* disagreed and reacted with undisguised emotion to the **NIH** decision, accusing the Consensus Conference of 'fraud' and 'condemning women to death'.[43]

Following political pressure from eight cancer organisations, five medical associations, and two US women's health organisations, the National Cancer Advisory Board (**NCAB**) reviewed the **NIH** judgement. Though both **NIH** and **NCAB** had access to exactly the same empirical evidence, **NCAB** chose an alternative emphasis. **NCAB** took the view that screening for the 40–49 year-old age group is likely to decrease mortality by around 17 per cent, and that the screening programme will save hundreds of lives annually (though **NCAB** confessed that the 17 per cent figure was based on only a few, limited scientific surveys). On March 27, on a vote of 17 for and 1 against, the National Cancer Institute (**NCI**) (**NIH**'s own cancer research wing) issued a **NCAB**-inspired recommendation in opposition to the **NIH** Conference, stating that women in their 40s at average risk of breast cancer should undergo mammography every one to two years.

Even though mammography is essentially a medical procedure subject to epidemiological assessment, there was clearly more than technical reason going on.

Spock-rationalists tend to see this sort of thing as an occasional blip, when the truth is that we combine reason and passion all the time. To give a further example: say you have a friend who's emigrated with his family to a foreign land after a great effort to get there, and yet a few months later he chooses to return home – at further great expense and the loss of his job – because he believes his teenage son will be happier. Economically, professionally and even socially all the calculations point to staying. But he can't. On the surface you might well judge your friend's behaviour irrational – but this would surely be a simplistic and unfair verdict. He loves his son so much, and the father/son relationship is so highly valued by him and his culture, that his emotional impulse rightly and rationally dominates.

IT IS IMPOSSIBLE FOR HUMAN BEINGS TO ACT IN VALUE-FREE WAYS

Some economists seem genuinely convinced that their profession is pure Spock-reason. They claim their role as economists is merely to provide the calculators, and that it is for others to say how they should be employed:

> '. . . is (it) appropriate or legitimate to use preferences of the community even if they can be successfully measured . . . (?) Certainly, as economists we would not claim that we can or should determine this but what we would want to investigate is whether the community has a view . . .'[44]

> 'Whose values should count? As a health economist it is not really for me to say. Nor, as a health economist, do I have to say . . .'[45]

> 'Is not the best researcher the "disinterested" researcher?'[46]

These Vulcans see themselves as field workers seeking merely to discover and respond to the wishes of the public. Yet any method of eliciting people's values will itself be based on values. The economist decides what area to investigate, what sort of questions to ask, who to ask, when to start and when to stop. The economist's method of calculation does not make these decisions for her – they are human choices beyond Spock-reason.

Take the example of opportunity cost ('opportunity cost' is the benefits one must forgo as one pursues a chosen goal: for example, a cost of my pursuing an opportunity to read a book to my daughters is not being able to work on my own book for a while). Health economists assume that because opportunity cost is an obvious truism, any application of it must also be unarguable. But this is like thinking that because we must all live on a planet where gravity is inescapable, any USE of gravity must be value-free. And this is blatantly untrue: anyone can see the moral difference between using sledges to slide injured people down mountain-sides and throwing children from tall buildings for sport.

This is not merely a theoretical problem. Every time health economists think they are doing something value-free when they are really making biased choices, they reinforce a technically obsessed health system. For example, a few years ago a team of health economists published an apparently innocuous paper[47] in which they described a project to obtain information from parents about child health services in Grampian region, North East Scotland. The economists chose to use a willingness to pay (**WTP**) method, as a way to elicit the parents' values (ironically **WTP** itself rests on the assumption that human decisions are driven first by values). They asked questions such as:

> 'Would you be willing to pay anything in extra taxation or a voluntary contribution for your child to receive day-case care instead of in-patient care?'

> 'What is the maximum amount that you would be willing to pay over the next 12 months for your child to receive day-case care instead of in-patient care?'

in order to discover the weight of parents' preferences for day-case surgery and overnight stay for tonsillectomy. They also tried to find out parents' preferences for hospital-based clinics and local clinics for bed-wetting, and school health services for all children and only for those with special needs.

The questions, they said:

> '... were framed in such a way as to provide realistic options to the parents'[46]

They also explained that:

> 'The questions reflected choices that the Health Board were [sic] making regarding how it should allocate the limited resources at its disposal between competing causes.'[46]

The economists maintained that they were merely carrying out a commission, in a disinterested way – as if they were mathematicians paid to provide a solution to an abstract numerical problem. But it just isn't so.

One need only ask them: would your research programme have been disinterested had the Grampian Board asked you to look into the following issues instead?

> Whether parents accused but not convicted of child abuse should be allowed to see their children at home or in the 'care institution'?

> Whether children should be fitted with electronic tags and tape-recorders and allowed home until the court case, or should always be accompanied by supervisors?

> Whether parents would prefer health service spending on child abuse investigations to be increased, or whether spending should be spread across all children?

In case the point is not already plain, one might ask a further question: would your research be disinterested if you were approached by a military regime interested in gaolers' preferences in regard to three sorts of torture? Presumably any economist would think very seriously about the hypothetical Grampian issues – both because these are sensitive matters and because each reflects a debatable way of spending public money. And presumably any honourable economist would refuse to entertain the army's request. But to concede this is plainly to admit that producing any results to meet specific 'information needs' cannot be value-free.

The Scottish economists might respond that there is a marked contrast between their actual project and the additional examples. But though there is an obvious difference in degree of controversy, they would be wrong to think there is a difference in kind. Let's spell it out:

- Deciding to take on the actual Grampian project was to decide not to do all those other things they might have been doing instead (opportunity cost). Some of those things they chose not to do must have been morally worse and some must have been morally better than doing what they did.
- To constrict their research programme as they did (which was admittedly the only way to meet the Grampian board's request) is to do research in an artificial box. It is to say: out of all the services on which parents might be asked to report their willingness to pay, we will inquire only about these. Thus the economists both accept the Grampian board's value-judgement (the board could have commissioned all manner of alternative projects) and make their own judgement that the research is worthwhile (just as they would doubtless judge the torture research not worthwhile).
- To accept this reality (the prevailing state of affairs in Grampian region) is to accept the status quo, which is a value-judgement regardless of whether you think you can do anything to change it (you don't have to choose to be part of it).
- To accept this reality is to accept the necessity of rationing in the areas on which questions were asked. Each question was an either/or, and gave parents no chance to say, for instance, 'we'd like to see tonsillectomy day surgery expanded *and* more provision for in-patient care'. Thus, by asking these questions the researchers cannot help but add to the climate in which this form of rationing is regarded as inevitable. Their research is – undeniably – a particular social intervention, based on a particular set of values and prejudices.

EVIDENCE AND VALUES ARE ENTWINED

The relationship between evidence and values is symbiotic. Without values we cannot discriminate between useful and useless evidence. Without evidence our preferences are uninformed.

EVIDENCE WITHOUT VALUES OR INTERPRETATION

Evidence is all around us. When we observe something without classification or preference, as a new-born does, we see evidence as purely as we humans are able to see it. Once we begin to learn classifications (for example, edible/inedible; pleasant/unpleasant; naughty/nice) we increasingly lose the ability to see the evidence in a neutral fashion. As we focus more and more on the evidence we want to focus on, we lose the ability to see the rest of the glorious cornucopia.[1]

VALUES WITHOUT EVIDENCE

If I believe that a person I know nothing about is a bad person because I don't like strangers, or if I've heard the mysterious word 'Pre-School' and yet decide not to go because I don't like mysteries, or if I believe the sun is a God, then I am valuing without any evidence – I am exhibiting a groundless prejudice and, if I am sensible, ought to go out and find some evidence to test out my values.

THE SPLIT BETWEEN REASON AND PASSION

Obviously evidence and values are entwined. Obviously all decisions are a balance of evidence and values. Obviously we should regard our values as at least equally important as evidence. And yet we don't.

It isn't particularly easy to understand why. We know we value. We know we are passionate creatures. And yet we want more and more evidence and less and less values in our decision-making.

Possibly the answer lies partly in what seems to be a dread of values (we don't deliberately create values, they happen to us, we have little or no power over them, and this disturbs us), and partly in the social legacy of a long series of scholarly attempts to separate reason and passion.

The history of philosophical thought is threaded through with debate about the relationship between emotion and reason.[48] It is impossible to review this momentous topic here. However, a little grounding will help show that far from being a fad, values-based decision-making (or **VDM**) is part of a continuing struggle to establish the balanced exploration of human creativity.

Thus, with apologies to students of **Philosophy 101** everywhere, here is an extremely brief review of the background to The Split.

PLATO'S THEORY OF FORMS

Plato categorised the universe into two parts: the perfect 'world of forms' and the imperfect 'world of appearance' (our physical habitat). According to Plato, the world of forms is reality as it REALLY is: eternal, unchangeable, and unknowable through sense experience (which can perceive only transient phenomena in the world of appearance). Knowledge gained from the world of Forms is infallible, whereas conclusions drawn from sensory experience are only ever probable to some degree. Human beings can achieve TRUE knowledge, but only through the exercise of reason.

Plato's idea is easiest to understand with reference to mathematical entities. A circle, for instance, is mathematically defined as a plane figure composed of a series of points, each of which is equidistant from a centre point. No one has ever seen a perfect circle (or 'the Form' of a circle, to use Plato's term) since it is not possible to create perfection in our imperfect world. It is impossible to draw a perfect circle with a pen because the circle will be distorted by flaws in the paper, the limitations of the pen, or the inadequacies of the human hand and eye. However, an object in the physical world may be CALLED a circle or a square or a triangle if it resembles (or 'participates in') the Form 'circularity', 'squareness' or 'triangularity'.

Although the Form of a circle can never be witnessed physically, mathematicians and others know for sure what a perfect circle is because they understand its definition. For Plato this implies that the Form 'circularity' must exist as a changeless object in the world of Forms, or else how could anyone know of it?

Plato extended his theory beyond mathematics. For example, he claimed that the word 'justice' can be applied to hundreds of different acts because these acts share in the

Form 'justice'. Similarly, an object is beautiful to the extent that it participates in the Form of beauty; an action is courageous or cowardly to the extent that it participates in the Form 'courage' or 'cowardice', and so on.

There is certainly something magical about Plato's idea. Everything in the world of space and time is what it is by virtue of its resemblance to its perfect, universal Form. We can use our minds to reach out to these sparkling eternal truths, even though we must inhabit a world of impermanence and illusion. We are chained to a shadowy reality but so long as we know how to look we can see beyond it – maybe we can even catch a glimpse of the mind of God.

Plato's distinction between appearance and reality is unquestionably compelling. Unfortunately, it has proven so persuasive to so many of us that it has played a large part in relegating our everyday world (the place where we feel, value and experience life) to second or even third class status.

To use a sporting analogy, Plato arranged reality and experience in three divisions:

PLATO'S DIVISIONS

Division One: Absolute truth (the eternal Forms) – can be reached by pure reason

Division Two: Science (uses both reason and physical evidence) – can come ever closer to absolute truth as its understanding of physical reality grows, but can never achieve certain knowledge because scientific inquiry does not take place in the world of Forms

Division Three: Passion and faith, art and poetry – the least real aspects, solely appearance, do not have eternal Forms. Plato went so far as to claim that art perverts and corrupts because it is nothing more than 'imitation' of an already imperfect world. According to Plato, art causes us to become attached to the wrong things – impermanent, shadowy, immoral things – rather than the eternal Forms.[49,50]

DESCARTES' SCEPTICISM

Echoing Plato's distinction between appearance and reality, René Descartes wondered how he could be sure any of his beliefs were true. Perhaps everything he perceived was really an illusion or a dream. Maybe God or an evil demon was trying to deceive him. How could he tell for sure?

In *Meditation 2*, Descartes thinks he finds a belief that is certainly true. Here's what he says:

> ...I have convinced myself that there is absolutely nothing in the world, no sky, no earth, no minds, no bodies. Does it not follow that I too do not exist? No: if I convinced myself of something then I certainly existed. But [suppose] there is a deceiver of supreme power and cunning who is deliberately and constantly deceiving me. In that case too I undoubtedly exist, if he is deceiving me; and let him deceive me as much as he can, he will never bring it about that I am nothing so long as I think that I am something. So after considering

everything very thoroughly, I must finally conclude that this proposition, I am, I exist, is necessarily true whenever it is put forward by me or conceived in my mind.[51]

We can imagine that our sense perceptions may be illusions, but it is impossible to doubt that we have minds, because the very process of doubting proves we have a mind to doubt with. By means of this analysis (and other arguments) Descartes promoted mind (or thinking) to Plato's **Division One** and left body (and the physical world) languishing in **Division Two**, or maybe **Division Three**.

According to Descartes the mind can know the beauty of mathematical relationships and that a supreme being exists. The body, on the other hand, is nothing more than a machine.

SPOCK'S ANXIETY IS OUR ANXIETY

We worry about our passions almost as much as Spock does. We think they are wild, instinctive, thoughtless, programmed by biology – we suppose they cloud our judgement.

Rational Plan (Good)	**The Split – the desire to disconnect reason from passion**	**Passionate Drive (Bad)**
Civilised Reasoned Thoughtful Intellectual activity and free will		Wild Instinctive Without thought Biological programming

Really Real	**Not So Real**
Analytic Truths (for example, mathematical proofs) (**Division One**) Mind/Intellectual Perception (**Division One**) Logic (**Division One**) Eternal Forms (**Division One**) 'I think therefore I am' (**Division One**)	Scientific Knowledge/evidence (**Division Two**) Body/Physical Perceptions (**Division Two/Three**) Emotion (**Division Three**) Opinion about the merit and use of scientific knowledge (**Division Three**) Art, poetry, music, creativity, passion, values (**Division Three**)

Innumerable thinkers and planners have shared Plato's distaste for the emotional side of human affairs. Most have come to Spock's conclusion that passion is an irrational blight, something to be defeated – a threat to human progress:

> The irrationalist insists that emotions and passions rather than reason are the mainsprings of human action...the rationalist repl(ies) that...we should do what we can to remedy (them)...[52]

Indeed, for Karl Popper, emotions and passions are no less than criminal tendencies:

> It is my firm conviction that this irrational emphasis upon emotion and passion leads ultimately to what I can only describe as crime...[52]

I share Popper's dislike of violence and the 'might is right' approach to human affairs. But it is much more difficult to see why – or even how – reason can be a remedy for our emotions and passions. How can reason be an antidote for something beyond reason? If passion and reason are completely separate, surely reason and passion cannot touch each other.

Even if a rational remedy for irrationalism were possible, what exactly should it remedy? Presumably not all emotions and passions are bad – otherwise Karl Popper's emotional aversion to violence and Plato's condemnation of poetry would be just as much precursors to crime as any other passionate judgement.

But if some passions are good and others bad, how are we to decide which are which? Can we define them in principle? Or should we define them only in accord with their effects?

We might say that as a rule envy is a bad passion, and always leads to bad consequences. But if we do, we must therefore appeal to an opinion about the nature of envy. And if we use examples to show that envy is destructive, then we must show that envy is NEVER a good thing, which is impossible to do.

This is not to deny that some emotions have bad consequences (envy usually does, in my experience). Nor is it to say that reason cannot be used to help us control our damaging emotions, both in personal life and in social policy-making. Clearly reason can and should do this: for example in the shape of well-drafted laws to control antisocial behaviour. But it is definitely to deny a special, privileged, Platonic place for reason. Reason is an aspect of us. It is not a dispassionate, God-like arbiter on permanent stand-by with completely objective solutions.

We will have arguments why we should respond to a fierce Klingon attack with equal hostility (Klingons are notorious enemies of Spock and his Starship Enterprise colleagues). Perhaps we will come up with logical ways to cause the Klingons as much hurt as possible. But we can't possibly make these deliberations according to Spock-reason alone. We may apply reason to work out the best strategies, but Spock-reason doesn't emerge spontaneously, in some emotional vacuum. We engage in them because our emotions have already told us what to feel.

It is easy to understand why we should fear the narrow-minded desires of emotionally stunted people who manipulate their way into political power, but the fact we fear or dislike their emotions is no reason at all to fear or dislike ALL emotions. Shouldn't we rejoice in being afraid of the behaviours of people we believe are misguided? It is our own emotional worlds that give us the freedom to despise them and the commitment to defeat them if we have to. It is because of our passions – and only because of them – that we can find the courage to challenge those things we find emotionally negative.

In sum, we might perhaps be right to fear all emotions if:

1. All emotion is bad
2. It is possible to select problems to solve without any emotional impetus
3. All problems are equal

But clearly none of these conditions is true. Not only is all emotion not a bad thing, it is very plainly necessary for any sensible problem-solving. Indeed, emotional impetus is necessary for any REASONABLE problem-solving: without emotion to guide our selection of problems we will either select problems to be solved arbitrarily, or we will pick them according to a totally rigid set of rules.

THE BIOLOGY OF HUMAN DECISION-MAKING

Resembling Vulcans in the way we idealise ourselves, we have got into the habit of regarding our emotional world as some sort of evolutionary deficit: emotions are bad; logic is good. And yet science itself shows us that we are wrong.

What may be true about the behaviour of an ant seeking out a cake crumb, or a surgeon expertly wielding a scalpel, is only a part of the story of human problem-solving drives:

> There is...considerable evidence...that the RH (right hemisphere of the brain) is essentially the seat of intuition, and that it thinks quite independently of the LH. One way of characterising intuitive thought is to say that, although it is logical, the standards of evidence it uses to make judgements are very different from the standards we normally associate with logical thought. In ordinary discourse, for example, when we say two things are the same, we mean they are identical in every respect; the standard of evidence we demand to justify such a judgement is extremely demanding. But when we construct a metaphor, e.g., the overseas Chinese are the Jews of the Orient, we pronounce two things to be the same in a very different sense...

> The history of man's creativity is filled with stories of artists and scientists who, after working hard and long on some difficult problem, consciously decide to 'forget' it, in effect, to turn it over to the RH. After some time, and often with great suddenness and totally unexpectedly, the solution to their problem announces itself to them in almost complete form. The RH appears to have been able to overcome the most difficult logical and systematic problems by, I would conjecture, relaxing the rigid standards of thought of the LH... The RH is thus able to hit upon solutions which could then, of course, be **recast** into strictly logical terms by the LH. We may conjecture that in children the communication channel between the two brain halves is wide open...that may be why children are so incredibly imaginative; e.g. for them a cigar box is an automobile one moment and a house the next. [Bold mine.][53]

Examining the biological elements of human thinking and behaviour (never mind the psychological and moral aspects) shows that there is much more to us than self-interested, logical goal-following. There are crucial biological elements to our selection of problems. We do not always respond like ant-automata to our environment, rather we are physically, mentally and socially disposed to select one problem or goal rather than another by factors which include our physical environment, drives and instincts, our social environment and history, and our personal preferences or values.

OUR PHYSICAL ENVIRONMENT, DRIVES AND INSTINCTS

There is no disputing that the physical environment stimulates our decision-making. If a rock falls from a cliff in front of the ant's path to a cake crumb the ant will respond by seeking an alternative route: if a radiator bursts in his car a human commuter will seek an alternative way of getting to work.

Neither is there any dispute that basic human needs stimulate our decision-making. We are driven to eat and drink to survive, we are drawn to sexual intercourse because we are somehow programmed to enjoy it (no doubt because this is the best way to ensure our propagation), we must confront or run away from danger, and so on. If we are hungry we make the decision to eat according to some combination of implicit bodily compulsion (I just *had* to eat some Tofu...), explicit desire not to be hungry, implicit desire for the most pleasurable taste available, ease of access to food, degree of risk associated with gathering food, and so on.

The ancient hunter stalking his prey with a spear was both physically driven and logical – when he needed food (a basic drive) he assessed the evidence in order to find the best way to get it. If a particularly desirable item of food looked hard and risky to obtain then the sensible hunter would, on balance, decide not to chase it if a less desirable item was plentifully and safely available.

Without doubt, as the hunter calculates the potential trade off between his ideal target with a low chance of success and a less desirable but acceptable option with a greater chance of success, he is engaging in an analysis beyond instinct, based on experience and intelligent understanding of probability. Nevertheless, even this more characteristically rational analysis is driven by his desire to eat safely. Without this desire there simply could not be any rational analysis at all.

These days we tend to think of this rational element as a means of controlling our rampant animal drives. The dieter, for example, really wants to eat but has decided to stick to a rational strategy to reduce his calorie intake. By dieting he seeks to use reason to control his instinct, which he treats with suspicion at best, and alarm and disgust at worst.

JOINED UP PEOPLE IN A JOINED UP WORLD

One of the most encouraging developments in recent years has been the growing recognition by neurobiologists that though we are biochemical beings, we are not merely logical processors fuelled and sustained by neurons and synapses. Rather we are logical and emotional creatures parcelled up as flesh, blood and reactions. Our physical drives and instincts have levels and subtleties that fundamentally undermine Simon's ant metaphor (see the **Introduction** to this book). Physical changes to our drives and environments, and to the ways our brains mediate our drives and environments, can fundamentally affect our problem-solving and goal-seeking behaviours in two important ways.

1. If our brains are damaged or our environments change, then our problem-solving capacities are also likely to change. If, for example, we are unfortunate enough to suffer a moderate stroke, we will not be able to solve as many problems as we would previously have done. We might, for instance, need to find other ways than speech to express our immediate needs. Equally, if we are confined to a hospital bed rather than our normal environment, some of our old problems (what shall I cook for dinner?) will have been superseded by new ones (how can I reach that pencil to try to write a message?).
2. More fundamentally still, changes in our brains and our environments (which we habitually and erroneously think of as separate) affect what occur to us to be problems and goals at all.

Both these phenomena are illustrated by Antonio Damasio's retelling of the strange case of Phineas Gage in his book *Descartes' Error*.[54]

Phineas Gage

Phineas Gage was a 'most efficient and capable man', a construction foreman in charge of blasting stone to construct a new railroad in Vermont in 1848. Gage suffered an accident in which a tamping iron (3 feet 7 inches long, one and a quarter inches in diameter tapering to one quarter inch) was blown through his left cheek, traversed the front of his brain, and exited at high speed through the top of his head to land over 100 feet away.

Amazingly, Gage recovered. He regained his physical strength. He could touch, hear, and see. He walked firmly, used his hands with dexterity and had no noticeable difficulty with speech or language. He could calculate just as well as ever. And yet, as his doctor recounted, the:

> ...equilibrium or balance, so to speak, between his intellectual faculty and animal propensities[55]

had been destroyed. He was now:

> ...fitful, irreverent, indulging at times in the grossest profanity which was not previously his custom, manifesting but little deference for his fellows, impatient of restraint or advice when it conflicts with his desires, at times pertinaciously obstinate, yet capricious and vacillating, devising many plans of future operation, which are no sooner arranged than they are abandoned...[55]

Damasio explains that:

> While other cases of neurological damage that occurred at about the same time revealed that the brain was the foundation for language, perception and motor function...Gage's story hinted [that]...somehow there were systems in the human brain dedicated more to reasoning than to anything else, and in particular to the **personal and social dimensions of reasoning**. The observance of previously acquired social convention and ethical rules could be lost as a result of brain damage, even when neither basic intellect nor language seemed compromised...[T]he alterations in Gage's personality were not subtle. He could not make good choices, and the choices he made were not simply neutral...one might venture that either his value system was now different, or, if it was still the same, there was no way in which the old values could influence his decisions...Gage lost something uniquely human, the ability to plan his future as a social being. [My bold][55]

Gage's intellectual reasoning was as able as ever – he was entirely rational in a logical sense – but he was emotionally and socially incompetent. He could readily approach problems according to the scheme in **Figure 1**, for example – but he was unable to select socially appropriate goals to pursue. Gage's ability to assess evidence was as good as ever, however his capacity for choosing which evidence it made social sense to assess had been fatally damaged by an accident to a part of his brain. Gage could no longer match his logic to his social contexts and so went from riches to rags, to die friendless and in poverty a few years after his catastrophe.

Building on the Gage case, Damasio outlines accumulating evidence that the intellect alone is not sufficient for us to manage the social world. Drawing on contemporary neuroscience, Damasio argues (against Descartes' error) that we are not conscious minds mysteriously separated from our unconscious bodies. Rather we think *somatically* – our bodily responses are *part of* our mental reactions to events. The parts of the brain necessary for balanced reasoning are the parts that connect our bodily responses to our emotional ones. And so our problem-solving and choice of problem to solve has both a logical and emotional basis:

> Imagine meeting a friend whom you have not seen for a long time . . . what happens to you, neurobiologically, as that emotion occurs? What does it really mean to 'experience an emotion'? . . . there is a change in your body state defined by several modifications in different body regions . . . your heart may race, your skin may flush, the muscles in your face change around the mouth and eyes to design a happy expression. . . . there are changes in a number of parameters in the function of viscera (heart, lungs, gut, skin) . . . .[56]

Damasio argues that:

> **The action of biological drives, body states, and emotions may be an indispensable foundation for rationality**. The lower levels in the neural edifice of reason are the same that regulate the processing of emotions and feelings, along with global functions of the body proper such that the organism can survive . . . Rationality is probably shaped and modulated by body signals, even as it performs the most sublime distinctions and acts accordingly. [Bold mine][57]

Human beings are not machines of technical reason. We do reason, but both what we reason about and the way we reason are profoundly and inextricably linked to our emotional experience of the world.

Damasio describes a 'somatic-marker', which we unconsciously experience as we make a choice about how to act:

> . . . the key components (of the choice in question) unfold in our minds instantly, sketchily, and virtually simultaneously, too fast for the details to be clearly defined. But now, imagine that *before* you apply any kind of cost/benefit analysis to the premises, and before you reason toward the solution of the problem, something quite important happens: when the bad outcome connected with a given response option comes into mind, however fleetingly, you experience an unpleasant gut feeling [Damasio calls this a somatic marker].

> What does the *somatic marker* achieve? It forces attention on the negative outcome to which a given action may lead, and functions as an automated alarm signal: Beware of danger ahead if you choose the option which leads to this outcome. The signal may lead you to reject, *immediately*, the negative course of action . . . allow[ing] you *to choose from among fewer alternatives*. There is still room for using a cost/benefit analysis and proper deductive competence, but only *after* the automated step drastically reduces the number of options.[58]

If you live in a large city and wish to go for a meal it would be absurd to start from scratch, analysing the pros and cons of every restaurant listed in the phone book. And of course no one does this because:

- It would take too long
- We have existing experiences of food and restaurants
- We have physical desires for certain types of food rather than other types

These desires can be stated explicitly ('You know what, I really fancy Thai tonight'), but they needn't be, because they are remembered by our bodies. And in exactly the same way, our choice of house, or friends, or leisure pursuit, or holiday, or disease therapy and so on is honed down for us by this somatic marker – amongst other social and logical influences. It quite clearly cannot be honed down for us by Spock rationality alone.

OUR SOCIAL ENVIRONMENT AND HISTORY

Damasio's commonplace examples of what it is like to experience an emotion reintroduce us to the obvious – they remind us that as our bodies react to an exciting situation, for example, we experience physical, emotional and conscious change all at once. Indeed, if you think of any everyday human experience, even the classifications 'physical', 'emotional' and 'conscious' are insecure. We have separate words and ideas for these categories (we even have separate disciplines that research and teach them) but are they REALLY separate? I think there is room for doubt.

The more exhilarating incidents illustrate the point best (though any human experience will do). For example, imagine attending a crowded soccer game where it matters intensely to you and everyone else around you that your team wins in order to avoid relegation. It's 0–0 and there are five minutes to go. You and everyone else have steadily become more and more despondent as the game has worn on. It looks like the boys won't score if they play until Wednesday week. Then your team flukes a corner. There's a goal-mouth scramble. The ball bounces tantalisingly out to your unmarked centre-forward. To everyone's astonishment, his shot rockets the ball into the top corner of the net. You spontaneously hug the stranger next to you. All you can hear are cheers, and all you can feel is heat and breath and jostling – at that moment you do not think of yourself as separate from anything. In fact you do not think of yourself at all – you are there physically *and* emotionally and it would be arbitrary to separate out the emotional bits from the physical ones. Your happiness *is* your experience and your experience *is* your happiness.

This essential interconnectedness (that we habitually deny as we classify reality) can be found in two forms in the Phineas Gage example. There is Damasio's interpretation that Gage's accident destroyed the part of the brain that links the 'somatic marker' to the part of the brain that processes emotions, and therefore disabled Gage's ability to act in a socially connected fashion. And there is the further point that Damasio's 'somatic marker' is not an independent thing either. Whether you have a pleasant or unpleasant experience as the result of a social behaviour depends both on the behaviour *and* its social context. Phineas Gage's changed behaviours were perceived as unwelcome by a social system that didn't value his uncompromising rationality. But a different system might conceivably have valued the changed Gage differently. He might, for example, have made an ideal mercenary soldier.

OUR PERSONAL PREFERENCES OR VALUES

To continue with the restaurant analogy, however our preferences are formed – through peer pressure, through biological conditioning, by our genes, by instinct, by our personal experiences, by intellectual analysis (by thinking about what we REALLY like) – it is quite certain that we DO have preferences. For whatever reason, we value some things more highly than others.

Talking about values is a useful way of summarising the above influences – for most purposes it doesn't matter how we got the values, what matters is that we do have them, that they influence our lives in all manner of ways, and that they influence the lives of the people who come into contact with us.

It is an awful mistake to separate logic and emotion as we do. Everybody accepts that environmental forces interact with our physical drives to form the problems and goals we face and choose; so why should we assume that our physical drives are somehow disconnected from our emotional ones? How could this even be? No one experiences life purely intellectually – so why on earth do we find it even remotely plausible to think of ourselves as human information processors alone?

> Be careful whenever a philosopher (or anyone) begins talking about 'reason' – just as when Mr. Spock used to say in *Star Trek*, 'Logic dictates.' Logic doesn't dictate very much, and we must be very careful what someone means by 'reason' when they begin invoking it...logic requires premises, and it ultimately cannot prove those premises. If 'reason' means logic, it really only means *consistency*; but in principle, there could be an infinite number of consistent logical systems...Hume...properly asserts that, 'Reason is and ought to be the slave of the passions.'[59,60]

CHAPTER TWO

The Dominance of Values

... value judgements are logically necessary for all decisions, so, irrespective of the amount of certainty and uncertainty in the scientific evidence, the most that scientists can do is *inform* values-based decision-making...

(Jack Dowie)[61]

SUMMARY

- The belief that problems come first is an illusion
- We must balance reason and emotion
- The only way we can hope to balance reason and emotion is to accept that values come first – to acknowledge once and for all that values dominate the evidence
- This is true of all human judgements, even those described as 'clinical'

◆

THE ILLUSION THAT PROBLEMS COME FIRST

Three misperceptions skew our view of the world and our place in it:

1. There are objective problems
2. We have no choice but to try to solve our objective problems
3. Our evaluative selves are in some way separate from our logical or intellectual selves

These ideas are everywhere, woven like tapestry into the very atmosphere of modern life. Nevertheless, each of them is mistaken.

THERE ARE NO OBJECTIVE PROBLEMS BECAUSE WITHOUT INSTINCTS, EMOTIONS AND VALUES THERE CAN BE NO PROBLEMS

Of course we encounter unexpected problems. And of course these problems are sometimes so overwhelming that we have to drop everything else to try to deal with

1st: Problems $\Longrightarrow$ 2nd: Instincts/needs/values (a reaction) $\Longrightarrow$ 3rd: Goals
(to solve the objective problem)

Figure 10

1st: Instincts/needs/values $\Longrightarrow$ 2nd: Goals $\Longrightarrow$ 3rd: Problems (if goals thwarted)

Figure 11

them. If we become ill, if we have a serious road traffic accident, if we experience a financial or existential crisis, then it can certainly seem as if our lives and decision-making are problem driven. In such circumstances things LOOK like **Figure 10**.

A problem hits Alan unexpectedly. He crashes his car on the motorway. He's injured, he hurts, he's scared, he's taken to hospital, he undergoes surgery, he spends weeks rehabilitating. He reacts to his problem emotionally and instinctively. He doesn't want the situation he finds himself in because it gets in the way of what he normally wants to do. It forces him to change his goals from the normal set to a set brought on by the accident.

Yet even in circumstances such as these, Alan's problems are actually driven by values (as in **Figure 11**).

SPOCK-BUBBLES

The best way to understand this is to see the motorway accident in the form of apparently free floating bubbles of Spock-reason, where **bubble A** is Alan's goal-directed behaviour before the accident and **bubble B** is his goal-directed behaviour after the accident.

As tempting as it is to see a motorway crash as a problem that would be a problem regardless of any values – it is crucial to remember that no bubble of Spock-reason can exist in its own right. In reality, Spock-bubbles are not free-floating, independent, objective entities – rather they are created by a combination of emotion, physical environment, social environment and history, physical drives, instincts and preferences, as we saw toward the end of **Chapter 1**.

In Alan's case, **bubble A** has come into being because of normal social conventions – because of the way things are in 2005 – because the bubble's creator, Alan, has instincts to succeed in various ways, and because he values work, family and travel.

So long as the road accident is not fatal, a different Spock-bubble, **bubble B**, simply has to pop into existence because Alan still has instincts, needs and values, and he still inhabits a physical and social environment. But of course Spock-bubble **B** does not appear *ex nihilo* either. No Spock-bubble does. The content of Spock-bubble **B** depends upon the surrounding conditions which bring it into being. In this case, Alan's will to survive, the social importance of medicine and family (if these were not part of his social environment Alan would probably not have the option of rehabilitation) and the value Alan places upon getting Spock-bubble **A** back.

A. Alan's goal-directed behaviour before the accident

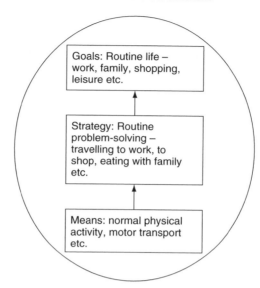

Figure 12

B. Alan's goal-directed behaviour after the accident

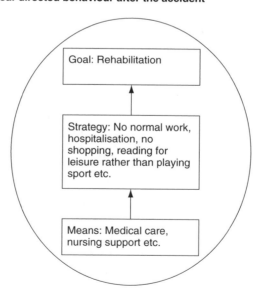

Figure 13

We almost always have a choice about which problems to solve

We have no choice but to try to solve SOME problems. Being alive MEANS having problems to overcome. But since there are no objective problems it is open to us – so long as we possess the freedom and imagination – to decide which challenges to take on and which to disregard.[1]

Our selves are both logical and emotional, and this affects all our judgements

It is only by coming to terms with this truth that we can hope to become more tolerant. Reason and emotion must be balanced.

WAR IS FOR REPTILES

All terrorists should be eliminated
Saddam Hussein is a terrorist
Therefore Saddam Hussein should be eliminated.

This is obviously a rational argument: if you believe your mortal enemy is a terrorist there is only one logical conclusion. Equally rational arguments proliferate in parliaments, news-media, bars and bus queues around the world. 'Why I Am in Favour of War.' 'Why We Must Overturn an Immoral Regime.' 'Why We are Right and They are Wrong.' But no matter from whom the arguments come, every one of them is beside the point.

Violent action is not rational. Yes, it can be wrapped about in rationality, but it does not originate from logically organised ideas. Anger, revenge and killing are irrationalities not because they cannot be argued, but because they are beneath reason. Such violences stem from fear, hatred and instinctive aggression. They are embodied emotion rooted in a time when syllogisms were unthinkable, but when there was war – a brute, natural war for the survival of species.

Neurobiology describes three anatomically distinct parts to the human brain. We share the most ancient with the reptiles and lower mammals, but the neocortex is specific to us. This human thinking cap – which enables us to use language, logic, and symbolic thought – has been superimposed on the primitive structures which control our biological drives and passions.

Unfortunately the 'wiring' connecting our 'three brains' seems to be faulty. As any one who has lost his temper knows, the neocortex cannot be relied upon to keep our instincts in check. Much worse, the neocortext is frequently unable even to recognise when the reptilian brain is in charge.

At the sniff of prey, the reptile brain dominates. Even though it cannot know their meaning, the reptile rejoices at the sound of grandiose arguments. 'Moral crusades', 'Holy Wars', 'moral imperatives', 'ethical invasions', 'justified killing', 'friendly fire': the more we recite rational nonsenses, the less chance of us noticing it pulling the strings.

Whenever the reptile takes over we become slaves to its belligerent drives, puppets of our biological past. We become obsessed with survival, paranoid about outsiders, mentally disarranged. We say one thing, and do exactly the opposite.

When individuals exhibit such blatantly incoherent behaviour we call them mentally ill and attempt therapies to help them regain control of themselves. And yet collective madness is cause for celebration: flag waving, marching songs and stirring curses at the evil enemy.

But if psychotic behaviour is a health issue for an individual human being, how much more of a health issue must it be for us all? Why do we go so crazy when we smell blood? Why do we instantly forget that the basis of moral action is compassion and human creativity? Why are we so willing to destroy members of our own species? Why do so many of us worship war? If it is the reptile within us causing us to turn away from civilisation, can we cage it?

We need answers to these questions, and we need them now. Instead of passing mock rational resolutions, the United Nations should join with the World Health Organisation to instigate a massive, multidisciplinary research programme into the causes of warlike behaviours. It is the most fundamental of public health problems and should be treated accordingly. I am serious. Our situation is serious. The reptile wants us to kill each other, and the time to stop him is running out.[62]

In the terrible circumstances described in the box above, the greatest problem is NOT that we are slaves to our passions and our reptilian brain (we are not entirely enslaved and many of our passions are not at all reptilian). Rather the problem is that we don't even SEE their influence on our logic – our logic appears to us to be pure and therefore entirely reasonable.

We can cage the reptile using logic and OTHER emotions and values (like love and compassion), but if we are to do this we have to see ourselves honestly and in balance – we have to see ourselves and our projects for what we and they truly are. We have to learn to see logic's source.

VALUES FIRST

It is very easy to prove the dominance of values.

We are supposed to believe policy-making proceeds like this:

Evidence First
Values Second

Spock's Mistake is even worse since it is:

Evidence First
Values Irrelevant

But policy-making can't possibly happen in either of the above forms. It must proceed like this:

Values First
Evidence Second

This truth can be seen everywhere: in government documents, in news bulletins, in daily conversation, as we decide how to spend our personal money, as we decide how to spend our days, as we decide how to interact with one another. Evidence is all around us, but evidence alone can never tell us what to do.

Imagine, for example, that the 'public health movement' has got around to thinking that warfare might be a public health issue. What should the movement's members do? Should they undertake research of some kind? Should they decide warfare is too controversial an issue for public health professionals to pursue? Should they resolve that war isn't a health issue? Should they act immediately to prevent warfare on the ground that bombing and shooting people is obviously not good for their health? Or should they see war as an opportunity to foster community spirit – and so promote health – within their own nation?

Whatever they decide they will need a plan:

Here is one possible **Plan A**:

PUBLIC HEALTH PLAN A

PUBLIC HEALTH SPECIALISTS SHOULD TRY TO PREVENT WARFARE

Because

- Warfare shortens lives and causes sickness and injury
- The medical treatment of war-related sickness and injury is expensive. Where such disease is treated by publicly funded medical services warfare incurs financial cost to the state
- Warfare destroys public health infrastructures, such as adequate nutrition, sanitation, and protection from physical and psychological assault
- Warfare uses up resources that would be better spent on improving public health
- Warfare leads to long-term trauma and incapacity, and so incurs public health costs for upwards of fifty years after a particular war is over
- Warfare is ugly, vicious, inhumane and unhealthy

PUBLIC HEALTH PROMOTERS SHOULD TRY TO PREVENT WARFARE BY MEANS OF ONE OR MORE OF THE FOLLOWING METHODS

- *Education* – soldiers and potential soldiers should be presented with comprehensive evidence about the health damage they do to themselves and others, and enabled to make free and informed choices about whether to fight, even if they are already in the army
- *Training* – anti-violence techniques and instruction should be offered and promoted by public health specialists wherever there is the potential for people come into conflict
- *Indoctrination* – anti-war propaganda should be widely distributed to counteract politicians' pro-war campaigns. It should be made plain that warfare is to be feared (horrible real life images should be used), and the huge profits that arms companies make as a result of their trade should be given maximum publicity – as black a picture as possible should be painted about the undesirable effects of warfare and the immorality of the weapons industry

---

- *Legislation* – war promotion should be banned; no guns, toy soldiers or any other toy that glorifies warfare should be allowed to be sold; armies should not be funded by the state; war-like talk in public places should be outlawed, soldiers and their families should be forced to bear the cost of all medical treatments made necessary by their fighting
- *Prohibition* – warfare should be outlawed altogether

Plan A is clearly intended to improve people's health, and contains a consistent Spock-bubble strategy. If you happen to agree with it, it will probably look obvious. It might even look like you could come up with it from WITHIN a Spock-bubble alone.

Can you say the same about **Plan B**?

PUBLIC HEALTH PLAN B

PUBLIC HEALTH SPECIALISTS SHOULD ENCOURAGE PEOPLE TO GO TO WAR WHEN THEIR NATION IS THREATENED BY TERRORISM

Because

- War helps eliminate terrorism, and terrorism is bad for health
- Promoting warfare helps the weapons industry employ more people (it is well known that unemployment is a public health issue)
- Recruiting young people to the national army increases their physical fitness, knowledge, discipline and future work skills. All these are clearly in the interest of the public health
- Warfare increases feelings of nationalism and people's sense of belonging – it is common knowledge that a sense of belonging is very important for health
- Warfare is sometimes enjoyable – soldiers and the general public get pleasure and excitement from warfare

PUBLIC HEALTH PROMOTERS SHOULD ENCOURAGE PEOPLE TO GO TO WAR WHEN THEIR NATION IS THREATENED BY TERRORISM BY MEANS OF ONE OR MORE OF THE FOLLOWING METHODS

- *Campaigning about the public health dangers of terrorism* – people could be made constantly vigilant for suspicious packages, vehicles and strangers. Particular attention could be paid to the medical dangers of bio-terrorism.
- *Campaigning about the personal and public health benefits of joining the army and/or supporting the war effort* – people could be encouraged to support war because their country needs them, and because they will feel a heightened sense of well-being and public spiritedness if they do
- *Setting up neighbourhood 'war support' schemes as a form of community development* – these schemes could bring like-minded strangers together and would also provide opportunities for more general health promotion and public health issue investigation

These two plans are deliberately provocative. They sound strange set side by side because most of us tend not to see warfare as a matter for public health work, and because we are not used to the idea of official bodies being so overtly partisan. Nonetheless, the underlying principle applies to any human plan, whatever its nature and whoever dreams it up.

Both plans are a combination of evidence *and* supposition, and neither is obviously the right public health approach (because there is no such thing as the obviously right public health approach). Both plans originate in alternative interpretations of the merits of warfare – neither plan is a neutral response to evidence, rather each is constructed according to this general formula:

Various pieces of evidence + Various sorts of opinion = A human plan[63]

VALUES-SOAKED PSYCHIATRY

Psychiatry offers a perfect real-world illustration of the above law. Psychiatrists often see the:

Values First
Evidence Second

reality as a problem for their profession. They would much rather hide behind a façade of medical objectivity. They would much rather have us believe they are dealing with solely evidence-based diseases and illnesses, the mental equivalent of broken legs and bacterial invasions, which would exist whether or not psychiatrists diagnosed them.

One can understand why many psychiatrists prefer to think like this, for otherwise they would be openly seen to be treating unusual human behaviours and thought patterns rather than clinical conditions. And yet – if you study psychiatry's diagnostic rule books – it is quite obvious that psychiatry rests on value judgement and value judgement alone, like this:

Values First
Diagnoses follow as a Consequence

To illustrate, the *Diagnostic and Statistical Manual of Mental Disorders* (4th edn) (DSM IV)[64] describes the following diagnostic criteria for 'Conduct Disorder':

> A. A repetitive and persistent pattern of behaviour in which the basic rights of others or major age-appropriate societal norms or rules are violated, as manifested by the presence of three (or more) of the following criteria in the past twelve months, with at least one criterion present in the past 6 months:
>
> **Aggression to people and animals**
>
> (1) often bullies, threatens, or intimidates others
> (2) often initiates physical fights
> (3) has used a weapon that can cause serious harm to others
> (4) has been physically cruel to people
> (5) has been physically cruel to animals
> (6) has stolen while confronting a victim (e.g. mugging, purse snatching, extortion and armed robbery)
> (7) has forced someone into sexual activity[65]

These 'clinical' criteria are blatantly evaluative. There is nothing technical or scientific about them whatsoever.

For example, deciding whether or not something is cruel is a moral judgement, inevitably influenced by social norms and conditioning. I believe that intensive farming of cattle for meat and dairy products is cruel to animals. Other people take a different view. If I were a psychiatrist assessing a cattle farmer's child for conduct disorder, should I include the child's enjoyment at herding cows into trucks heading for the slaughter house as indicative of criterion (5) or not? If a meat-eating psychiatrist from a pastoral farming family were to assess the child, what should he decide? Whether or not the child is diagnosed as 'cruel' depends solely on a value judgement about the behaviour.

Deciding whether 'often initiating physical fights' is a sign of psychological morbidity depends on whether or not you think such behaviour is admirable. If you live in a brutal neighbourhood you might be pleased to find your child exhibiting such strength of physique and character. It also depends on context. For example, if the initiation of physical fights is a child's response to bullying, a value judgement beyond the DSM IV criteria is immediately necessary – is it better to stand up to bullies or to take bullying on the chin? Indeed, is bullying itself a good or bad thing? It doesn't overtax the imagination to see bullying as good practice for a future as a political or military leader.

DSM IV tells us that it is possible to diagnose people over the age of 18 as having 'conduct disorder'. This being so, it is hardly stretching a point to say that George Bush and Donald Rumsfeld's behaviour toward the people of Iraq in 2003 and 2004 defines them as having conduct disorder according to the above criteria. Add:

> (8) has deliberately engaged in fire setting with the intention of causing serious damage
> (9) has deliberately destroyed others' property (other than by fire setting)
> (10) has broken into someone else's house, building or car
> (11) often lies to obtain goods or favours or to avoid obligations (i.e., 'cons' others)[65]

and there is surely a bullet-proof psychiatric case for a clinical intervention.

All this is embarrassingly, risibly obvious. Psychiatric diagnoses depend upon value judgements because psychiatric diagnoses are always verdicts about the desirability of human thoughts and actions.[66] It is remarkable (and very disturbing) that the biopsychiatry profession will not accept this reality. Presumably they are afraid that admitting it will undermine their status as a scientifically based profession, when in fact honesty always strengthens science. It would be perfectly reasonable and admirably frank to say, 'we do not like psychotic behaviour, which is why we have INVENTED diagnostic categories for it' AND to research possible biochemical causes and treatments. It would also be helpful if they were to admit that preference for biochemical explanations is evaluative too. They need not be too anxious about confessing this since it is true of any preference for any technological solution to any perceived problem.

There is a slightly more subtle point. DSM IV also makes a value judgement when it stipulates that conduct disorder:

> . . . is manifested by the presence of three (or more) of the following criteria in the past twelve months, with at least one criterion present in the past 6 months[65]

Why three criteria? Why not two? This isn't a matter of evidence, it's a matter of human choice. Why do two categories not count as conduct disorder, say:

> (6) has stolen while confronting a victim (e.g. mugging, purse snatching, extortion and armed robbery)
> (7) has forced someone into sexual activity

while:

> (6) has stolen while confronting a victim (e.g. mugging, purse snatching, extortion and armed robbery
> (7) has forced someone into sexual activity

plus

> (1) often bullies, threatens, or intimidates others

do count?

Disregarding the patently absurd elements involved in counting up lists of general, context-free statements about 'good and bad' behaviour, there is clearly a value judgement involved in choosing how many criteria to include as indicative of a 'mental condition'.

DSM IV has this to say about 'clinical judgement':

> It is important that DSM IV not be applied mechanically by untrained individuals. The specific diagnostic criteria included in DSM IV are meant to serve as guidelines to be informed by clinical judgement and are not meant to be used in cookbook fashion. For example, the exercise of clinical judgement may justify giving a certain diagnosis to an individual even though the clinical presentation falls just short of meeting the full criteria for the diagnosis as long as the symptoms that are present are persistent and severe.[67]

It is enormously difficult to see psychiatry as a clinical, evidence-based profession when a psychiatrist can use her 'clinical judgement' to decide that someone is mentally ill EVEN IF she is healthy according to the official rules.

DSM IV refers to 'clinical judgement' as if it is something that applies only to marginal cases, and rests primarily on clinical rather than social experience. To see that this is baloney, consider two psychiatrists – Lucy and Kate – whose judgment as clinicians is informed by different ways of looking at the social world in general, and at childhood in particular.

USING VALUES TO DIAGNOSE AD/HD

Lucy is in her early thirties and has no children. She was an only child and spent her early years on an isolated farm in beautiful countryside in the South Island of New Zealand. From the age of six she was very interested in poetry, and had written her own book of poems by her ninth birthday. Lucy liked to wander to favourite spots on the farm – a waterfall, a hill with distant views, an ancient tree with sweeping boughs. She would spend hours alone, dreaming of the adventures, loves and tragedies of imaginary characters.

Lucy did not do well in school. It was only on attending university as a twenty-one year old that she sprang to life academically. She has now found her vocation as a child psychiatrist.

Kate is 50 and comes from a strict Methodist background in Nottingham, England. From an early age she was taught obedience and Christian virtue, teachings she accepted without question. Kate lived happily at home until she left university; she was a member of the Young Conservatives and holds 'old-fashioned' views about personal discipline and self-control. Kate has never married, but has nieces and nephews. She is professionally fulfilled as consultant child psychiatrist.

Marjorie Smith – the mother of a ten-year-old child, **Terry** – brings her daughter to see Kate. Kate takes a history and decides that Terry fits criteria (1) a, b, c, d, e, f, h and i, and (2) a, b from the list of 'Diagnostic criteria for Attention-Deficit/ Hyperactivity Disorder' below. She tells Marjorie that Terry certainly has AD/HD.

Marjorie is alarmed to hear this. She makes an appointment for the following week, when Kate happens to be on holiday. Lucy sees her and Terry instead. She makes her own assessment of Terry. Lucy can see why Kate chose the categories she did but nevertheless reduces this list to (1) a, b, c, and (2) a from the list of criteria below. She tells Marjorie that this means that Terry is NOT AD/HD.

Diagnostic criteria for Attention-Deficit/Hyperactivity Disorder

A. Either (1) or (2):

(1) six (or more) of the following symptoms of **inattention** have persisted for at least six months to a degree that is maladaptive and inconsistent with developmental level:

Inattention
(a) often fails to give close attention to details or makes careless mistakes in schoolwork, work or other activities
(b) often has difficulty sustaining attention in tasks or play activities
(c) often does not seem to listen when spoken to directly
(d) often does not follow through on instructions and fails to finish schoolwork, chores, or duties in the workplace (not due to oppositional behaviour or failure to understand instructions)
(e) often has difficulty organizing tasks and activities
(f) often avoids, dislikes, or is reluctant to engage in tasks that require sustained mental effort (such as schoolwork or homework)
(g) often loses things necessary for tasks or activities (e.g., toys, school assignments, pencils, books or tools)
(h) is often easily distracted by extraneous stimuli
(i) is often forgetful in daily activities

(2) six (or more) of the following symptoms of hyperactivity impulsivity have persisted for at least 6 months to a degree that is maladaptive and inconsistent with developmental level:

Hyperactivity
(a) often fidgets with hands or feet or squirms in seat
(b) often leaves seat in classroom or in other situations in which remaining seated is expected
(c) often runs about or climbs excessively in situations in which it is inappropriate (in adolescents or adults, may be limited to subjective feelings of restlessness)
(d) often has difficulty playing or engaging in leisure activities quietly
(e) is often 'on the go' or often acts as if 'driven by a motor'
(f) often talks excessively

Impulsivity
(g) often blurts out answers before questions have been completed
(h) often has difficulty awaiting turn
(i) often interrupts or intrudes on others (e.g., butts into conversations or games)[68]

Marjorie is greatly relieved to hear this. Encouraged, Lucy tells Marjorie and Terry not to worry – not all children are the same and some children have fewer social interests than others. She asks if Terry enjoys writing stories and drawing pictures. Terry says this is her favourite thing to do. Lucy invites her to come to see her again in a couple of weeks and to remember to bring her stories. In return, Lucy promises to show Terry the book of poems she wrote as a little girl.

Both psychiatrists have looked at the evidence and both have exercised their clinical judgement – which is no minor matter to the lives of Terry and Marjorie.

Values are obviously everywhere, and yet we repeatedly ignore them and sometimes even try to cure ourselves of them. Why do we find our values such a challenge? How might we use values' constant presence to our collective advantage instead?

In order to answer these (and many other) questions, we need to examine the big picture.

PART TWO

The Big Picture

The Truth about Relativism

If a lion could talk, we could not understand him

(Ludwig Wittgenstein)[69]

SUMMARY

- Three apparently puzzling case studies are presented
- The problem of relativism is introduced – does values-based decision-making (**VDM**) imply relativism?
- The relationship between evidence and non-evidence is explored
- The notion of rational fields is explained
- The post-modernist folly over relativism is discussed
- The truth about relativism is revealed
- It is suggested that **VDM** may be an antidote to relativism
- The three case studies are briefly revisited in order to show how Wittgenstein's' mythical lion can be understood

Chapters One and **Two** have established that technical rationality has surprisingly narrow limits, and is always and everywhere dominated by human values. This conclusion is both obvious and disconcerting – we know the truth of it but somehow we don't want to accept our power to reinvent the social world.

Chapter Three describes the relationship between values and technical rationality in more detail, and attempts to deal with the BIG OBJECTION to values-based decision-making – namely that **VDM** implies that it is impossible to establish that any belief is better than any other belief. This objection is not true – it is undoubtedly possible to show that all sorts of ideas and policies are better or worse than others in all sorts of ways. However, it IS impossible to prove that anyone's values are objectively right or wrong.

Chapter Three also briefly explores Wittgenstein's famous dictum: 'If a lion could talk we could not understand him'. Once you understand how Spock-bubbles come into being, you can begin to explore all manner of routes into the lion's world, and can also consider all manner of ways of inviting the lion into your own.

If there is any merit in this idea at all, then **VDM** offers a hugely exciting prospect for greater tolerance and understanding between human beings.

◆

THREE CASE STUDIES

To begin with, consider three apparently unrelated situations:

THE SHELL PICTURE

Picture an artist walking absorbed along a sunny, blustery beach one day in early autumn. Her jade-coloured coat is open, billowing like a sail in her wake. The sea is foaming with white caps, but she hardly notices them. She is looking down, alternately frowning and smiling, occasionally bending to place a shell in a large basket.

The artist wants to make a picture from the shells. She is carefully selecting the most beautiful shells she can find. Satisfied, eventually, she lays the wet shells down in a glinting pattern on the sand. Now she smiles broadly. She shouts her friend over.

'I've done it. I love it. Look at my beautiful shell picture. I call it *Glory*', she says.

But her friend is mystified. All he can see is a pale, windswept beach with shells everywhere.

THE HARBOUR BRIDGE

Imagine the maritime city of Safe Harbour. Traffic congestion is getting out of hand. There are vehicles everywhere, crawling, speeding, rumbling, polluting. At peak times it's taking commuters almost half an hour to cross the pivotal harbour bridge. The council authorities have debated how to deal with the problem for years, and still haven't reached an agreement.

Recently, through a combination of commuter frustration, media pressure and campaigning by a bridge construction company, the need for an additional bridge has begun to dominate debate. Consultant engineers have been brought in to calculate the relative efficiencies of different bridge types, accountants have created spreadsheets to compare costs, risk-assessors have factored in safety standards, and councils have circulated newsletters and run focus groups to establish citizen preference.

Right at this moment it's a typical Monday morning. A stranger is standing at the top of the bridge. Because he's never been to Safe Harbour, he's elected to take the guided harbour bridge tour. He has the morning paper in his hand. Its banner headline reads 'Bridge Decision Today', but he has no interest in the story. Instead he stands, leaning into the refreshing breeze, both hands on the safety rail, with others in the group. He is transfixed by the sparkling harbour waters which stretch as far as he can see, between islands, into bays and beaches. In his mind's eye he sees a network of canals stretching into the heart of the city itself. 'So beautiful. So much possibility,' is all he can say.

THE EXPERT PANEL

A large table stands in the centre of an oak-panelled hall. Fifteen men and women are sitting around it. One man is very young – aged about 22 – the rest are middle-aged at least: a couple of them must be approaching retirement. They are deep in conversation.

MIDDLE-AGED WOMAN COMMITTEE MEMBER: Then we're agreed. For the Mid-Counties Merged University we will accept 85 per cent of their internal staff rankings but change the rest?

MIDDLE-AGED WOMAN COMMITTEE MEMBER 2: That is in line with our equity policy. We must be seen to treat all applicant universities even-handedly.

MIDDLE-AGED MALE COMMITTEE MEMBER: Apart from the Big Two, remember?

MIDDLE-AGED WOMAN COMMITTEE MEMBER 2: Of course, of course. Christfields and Victoria are our leading research institutions. They are, truth be told, our only universities of international standing and we must therefore look to maximise their PBRF ratings.

MIDDLE-AGED MALE COMMITTEE MEMBER: Quite so. We must use our expertise to determine the ranking of the less experienced institutions in the sector, while of course respecting the standing and authority of their Vice Chancellors.

ELDERLY MALE COMMITTEE MEMBER: So let's begin to mark down the worst 15 per cent from the newer universities. I think we should start with Tourism and Hotel Studies, don't you?

Amused guffaws and sniggers.

ELDERLY MALE COMMITTEE MEMBER: (*continuing mirthfully*) Of course I need to ask if anyone has a problem with that.

More sniggers.

ELDERLY MALE COMMITTEE MEMBER: Good. In that case I'd like to suggest that we reduce the grade for Professors Theroux and Le Roux from an A (international researcher standing) to a B (national researcher standing) and reduce the grade of Associate Professor Joy Wednesday-Shift RN from an A to a C....

YOUNG MAN: (*coughing, a little embarrassed*) Um, excuse me...

MIDDLE-AGED WOMAN COMMITTEE MEMBER 3: Aha! Our student representative for this week. How can we help?

STUDENT REPRESENTATIVE: It's...ah...well...look, the thing is...I'm sorry but I'm not following this at all.

MIDDLE-AGED WOMAN COMMITTEE MEMBER 3: (*over her reading glasses*) I see. What don't you understand? I would have thought it was quite clear what we're doing. We are assessing our universities' self-reported grades in the PBRF. You know, the Performance Based Research Funding exercise? The one we copied from the UK Research Assessment Exercise?

Silence.

MIDDLE-AGED WOMAN COMMITTEE MEMBER 3: And we're doing this so we can distribute government research funds fairly and in accord both with past merit in research and future promise in research. Would you like to ask a question?

STUDENT REPRESENTATIVE: I don't understand.

MIDDLE-AGED MALE COMMITTEE MEMBER 2: (*impatiently*) Tut, tut. What, precisely, do you not understand, young man?

STUDENT REPRESENTATIVE: (*riled*) Any of it. I don't understand anything about this.

MIDDLE-AGED MALE COMMITTEE MEMBER 2: Weren't you briefed?

STUDENT REPRESENTATIVE: I was, but I didn't get that either.

The committee members look mystified, in a patronising way.

STUDENT REPRESENTATIVE: (*taking a deep breath*) I reckon I appreciate what you think you are supposed to be doing, but I don't see how you can do it in any meaningful way. The PBRF exercise is costing millions of dollars even though everyone knows the universities that got the funding in the past will get the funding in the future. There simply can't be any other result because that's the way the PBRF exercise is set up. And at the same time most students will have to work for years and years just to pay back our loans. I don't see how it makes sense.

MIDDLE-AGED WOMAN COMMITTEE MEMBER 2: (*irritated*) Really. You don't understand? Well, dare I suggest that this is because this has got nothing to do with student issues? We're here to decide who's been doing the best research, not what to do about student loans.

STUDENT REPRESENTATIVE: But you already know who's doing the 'best research'. You just said so. The Big Two.

MIDDLE-AGED WOMAN COMMITTEE MEMBER 2: Of course. Goes without saying. But we need to undertake due process and assess the relative citation rates of each institution's academics...

STUDENT REPRESENTATIVE: Citation rates?

MIDDLE-AGED WOMAN COMMITTEE MEMBER 2: That's the amount of times an academic paper is referenced in other academic papers.

STUDENT REPRESENTATIVE: But what if some are praised and others criticised?

MIDDLE-AGED WOMAN COMMITTEE MEMBER 2: We consider that irrelevant to the assessment.

STUDENT REPRESENTATIVE: Why?

MIDDLE-AGED WOMAN COMMITTEE MEMBER 2: We made that decision. It is part of our baseline.

STUDENT REPRESENTATIVE: Why? How?

MIDDLE-AGED WOMAN COMMITTEE MEMBER 3: Look. This is all very interesting...a potentially stimulating debate in fact. And we thank you for it, really we do. But you must excuse *us* now. We have important matters to resolve and a pressing deadline to meet...

At first sight these three cases may seem puzzling and unrelated. Yet by the time you have read this chapter their meaning and relevance will be quite obvious. As they come into focus you will recognise the truth about relativism, understand the relationship between Spock-reason and values, and appreciate how **VDM** has the potential to liberate us from narrow-minded views of the world.

WHAT IS THE PROBLEM OF RELATIVISM?

In order to argue that values and evidence should be seen in proper balance, it is necessary to confront the problem of relativism, and in particular the problem of moral relativism.

Relativism is a significant topic of academic study, most notably within the philosophy of science, sociology, anthropology and moral philosophy. At its most general, relativism holds that there can be no such thing as absolute truth in any field of human enquiry.

According to relativism, all understandings of the external world – even in science and mathematics – are filtered through human perceptions and interpretations. Relativists say that it is impossible to step outside these human filters in order to comprehend truth or reality 'in the raw'. All we can do is accept the interpretations for what they are – ideas which make sense within the tradition that holds them, but which may not make sense within other traditions. Thus, if one social tradition tells us people get sick because of evil spells and another tells us people get sick because of toxic microbes, we have two choices. Either we can accept the view of one of the traditions, or we can reject the view of both and come up with an alternative we like better. But we cannot detach ourselves from our culture or era – we cannot step out of our particular view of the world in order to find out the REAL answer.

TYPES OF RELATIVISM

Academics describe different types of relativism.

Conceptual relativism maintains that our understanding of the world depends on the 'conceptual grid' through which we view it:

> ...different schemes of classification incorporate witches and tree spirits, phlogiston and the ether, electrons and magnetic fields .... Schemes of concepts provide grids on which to base belief...[70]

The idea is that the set of concepts in our individual grids create and limit the worlds we each see. If your conceptual grid does not include the concept 'electrons' you will be unable to see the world in the way a modern physicist sees it. If there is no place for 'witchcraft' within your grid of concepts you cannot possibly understand how spells can affect the future. And if you have no notion of 'mercy' you will either be mystified as you witness a merciful act, or you will translate that act in some other way, in accordance with the concepts in your particular conceptual grid.

Truth relativists take a similar line to the conceptual relativists:

> . . . what is true for the Hopi is not so for us; what is true for Aristotle is not true for Galileo . . .[71]

I recently experienced something like these forms of relativism. I was sitting in a queue at traffic lights, very late for class. The vehicles ahead were moving much more slowly than usual, and as a consequence I was becoming frustrated. When I eventually reached the front of the queue I saw that a car had broken down in one of the two available lanes. Just as I was about to pass the immobile vehicle and go through the light – which was on green – the car ahead of me pulled up beside it. To my shame I cursed and moaned, 'What the *$%$###! do you think you're doing!' Then I realised that the driver was winding down his window. He was talking to the woman, obviously asking if she needed any help. It turned out she did; and I had a salutary reminder about life's priorities. I experienced a powerful, almost other-worldly, effect of jumping from one frame of reference to another: at one moment I was impatiently focused on getting to a single destination, seeing everyone else as an obstacle; the next I was able to see a person in need and a kindly act. My outlook on the world changed in an instant.

Advocates of the **relativism of reason** go even further than the conceptual and truth relativists. For them, even the way we assess evidence and decide strategy is relative:

> . . . what counts as a good reason may be context-dependent. Galileo consulted observation and experiment, Bellarmine the scriptures; Evans-Pritchard the available evidence of causal connections, Azande the poison oracle. Each is equally enmeshed in a web of reasons, properly woven by its own standards from within but finally incapable of support from without.[72]

According to the **reason relativist**, not only are we unable to access truth independent of our human limitations, we cannot even be sure which methods to use to try to get closer to it.

There are several reasons to resist each of these forms of relativism, some of which are considered in passing later in this chapter. However, it is much harder to come to terms with **moral relativism**, which is the view that what is morally right or wrong is nothing more or less than whatever is held to be morally right or wrong by any particular group of people.

Many moral relativists go so far as to say that what is morally right and wrong is nothing more than what any particular INDIVIDUAL asserts. According to them, if Ann thinks disciplining children frequently with a hard stick is moral and Susan believes all forms of violence are unethical, it is impossible to appeal to an independent morality to arbitrate between them. Furthermore, neither Ann nor Susan can say anything to the other to convince her that her view is morally mistaken. The very best they can do is agree to differ.[73]

Moral relativism's challenge to VDM

Moral relativism poses a significant challenge for advocates of values-based decision-making. Why bother to make values transparent if there's nothing to choose between any of them? What does it matter if people choose one set of values rather than another? I may believe my values are superior to yours, but what use is that if I can't prove it? If all values are equal how can I plausibly condemn violence, or warfare, or gratuitous cruelty?

At first sight it seems as if values-based decision-making must either promote a single set of values as the RIGHT values, or be forced to concede that all values are equal.

Moral relativism is difficult to accept

Although it is obviously true that there is no morality independent of human choice, it is exceedingly hard for any of us to admit that our cherished moral outlook is no better than anyone else's.

Kim Woodbridge and Bill Fulford, themselves advocates of values-based practice, take the bull by the horns:

> Faced with the complexity of different people's values, we . . . feel . . . inclined to ask, 'But, who is right?' Much . . . ethical regulation (codes and guidelines) is based on prescribing 'right' values . . . if someone can tell us who is right . . . we feel we know what to do . . .[74]

They concede that:

> Of course, there is no such thing as 'right and wrong' . . .[74]

then immediately (and understandably) retrench:

> . . . (but) there are limits beyond which many of us would not be prepared to go . . . we will call (these) 'framework values' . . .[74]

Woodbridge and Fulford argue that there are no right values, and yet most of us are nevertheless aware of moral limits beyond which most people will not go. It is not at all clear how this can be so, but I have every sympathy for the authors' ambivalence. The implication that there are no moral rights and wrongs can be very hard to swallow. To accept it is also to accept that one cannot say with any objective authority that the attack on the World Trade Centre in 2001 was morally wrong.[75] Nor can one finally establish the moral wrongness of the values which motivated rebels in Beslan to slaughter scores of innocent children in 2004.[76]

It is very important to face this point head on. However much one may be sickened by the merciless killing of children and other citizens going about their daily business, no one can PROVE that these behaviours stem from indubitably bad values. As Woodbridge and Fulford note, in science there is often only one right answer, an answer that can be shown to be right regardless of what anyone believes (how fast light travels, for example) whereas in ethics there is always a range of views – and therefore always the possibility of plausible dissent.

Not everyone is appalled by violent behaviour against children and other civilians. Those of us who are can either say its perpetrators have the wrong values, or are mentally ill and therefore unable to reason morally correctly. Yet however we couch our criticism we still have to demonstrate that it is we who have the truly right values, and this just cannot be done.

IS THIS ALL WE CAN DO?

We can say we do not approve of behaviours and values that repel us, and we can point out reasons why other people should not approve of them either. Even though we cannot appeal to objective morality we can be passionately opposed to wanton cruelty. We can try to explain that the behaviour has detrimental consequences for all of us, or that it will ultimately be bad for its perpetrators, or that it is inconsistent with other behaviours and desires favoured by the perpetrators (like being kind to their own family or tribe, for example). We can also explain alternatives, but still we cannot prove that these alternatives are right *per se*.

It is hard to accept that this is all we can do. It is much easier to deny it, as I have done in the past.

How my distaste for moral relativism caused me knowingly to put forward a weak argument

I stoutly resisted moral relativism for years. In *Ethics: The Heart of Health Care*[77] I claimed that there is something absolutely immoral about deliberately restricting human potential – I labelled all such behaviours forms of 'dwarfing'. My argument was that:

> ... discover(ing) clear examples of morality (is) a false hope, but a solid base for ethical practice (can be) unearthed nevertheless.

> The problem with the ambition to find 'the truly moral' is that people hold beliefs and values whose truth or falsity cannot be objectively assessed. The statement 'water boils at 100 degrees Celsius at sea level' is testable. It can be shown to be true provided the definitions included in it, and the method of testing, are agreed. But the statement 'it is right to perform euthanasia on a patient who has repeatedly requested it' cannot be tested. It may be possible to establish how many times and under what conditions the patient expressed the wish, but it is impossible to discover experimentally whether or not a health worker would be morally right to assist ...

> It is an error to expect moral philosophy to come up with a set of statements – some sort of Midas formula – that will always turn a tough dilemma into a golden solution. A more achievable aim of ethical exploration is the clarification of thinking, arguments and problems, the disclosure to decision-makers of the full range of possibilities open to them, and the elucidation of different points of view and ways of reasoning.

> No moral rule exists that cannot be justifiably broken ... we can now begin to understand that although moral judgement has an essentially subjective component, this does not mean it is impossible to base moral principles on objective evidence.[78]

So far so good. However, this hopeful argument soon enters Indian country:

> Let us see how this can be so. The moral quality of actions depends at least in part upon the value of what they bring about. In order to know whether some action is morally good it is therefore necessary to understand what is worthwhile in two factual senses:
>
> i) It is necessary to understand what the people you will affect with your actions value (their values are subjective but *that* they value as they do is a fact).
> ii) It is necessary to understand that people do not have infinite potential, though they can develop in a wide range of ways. Some of these ways (continuing to breathe, not being in excruciating pain, being able to think) are absolutely necessary if they are to develop at all further. And some other ways (not being injured, not being seriously ill, not being ignorant) are necessary if their further development is to be fulfilling.

> Moral actions must intend to promote what is good in one or both of these senses, though how to do this specifically for the best must be the subject of careful deliberation in each case.[79]

In short, I was arguing that to qualify as moral, any action must respect the values of other people and/or support the achievement of their fundamental human potentials (or at least not inhibit them). Having 'established' this I went on to argue that:

> Work for health is a fundamentally moral endeavour because it encourages both biological and chosen human potential. Work for health is work to enable in both factual senses…point ii) (above) roughly has to do with *creating autonomy*, while point i) is concerned with *respecting* it.

> This insight undermines the is/ought objection. Being human and possessing a range of worthwhile potentials is a fact which contains an ought. That is, the statement 'Fred is a human being' contains within itself the statement 'Fred ought to be a human being'. This cannot be denied without absurdity.[79]

My simple (simplistic?) idea was that unless we are to deny completely the value of humanity we must uphold its purpose. And given that humanity's essential purpose is to act – to do – then we should, as a matter of both morality and health, ensure that as much fulfilling action as possible is brought into being.

I tried to reinforce this idea by proving that 'dwarfing' is intuitively immoral:

> Because there is a baffling variety of candidates for the title 'truly moral' and no uncontroversial criteria for judging between them, it is sensible to attempt to identify *immoral* actions in order to cast new light on their apparently polar opposite – the moral…

> Does a good parent leave his child in the care of others for long periods? Is the person who has little feeling for her child yet still provides diligently for all material necessities a good parent? Or does a good parent love her child so deeply that she will never let him out of her sight? It is hard to say which parent comes closest to 'the ideally good parent' because this label is so obviously contestable. However…although there is endless controversy about the definition of 'good parent', it seems possible to reach universal (or almost universal) agreement about what a bad parent is. For example, it would be very difficult to find a social worker who does not agree that a person who consistently and deliberately inflicts physical and mental harm upon her child, who never considers what might be good for him, and does not intend to produce long-term good either, is a bad parent…

The way of things in Grand Thiam

> Grand Thiam is a human civilisation [in] which…[D]espite enviable material wealth its residents are becoming vociferous: demanding power, demanding greater liberty, and demanding the right to decide their own destinies.

> This pressure for change is a serious threat to the government's priorities. Grand Thiam is ruled by 100 Elders not allowed to marry or procreate, but who can select their successors without public consultation. For them the ideal society has strong social cohesion, every citizen knows his place in it, there is unquestioning obedience to the law, all industry is able to achieve maximum productivity, and disease is kept to a minimum. They prefer these values over such alternatives as free and uncensored speech, public participation in decision-making, and equal opportunity of access to political power. From the Elders' point of view, the more such values proliferate the more the *status quo* is threatened.

> Through a recently developed cocktail of genetic and educational manipulation the Elders now have the power to engineer their perfect world.

Dwarfing

> Time has moved on and the Elders have used the technology. The 'educational' part of the process made use of a Platonic 'noble lie'. All history books were destroyed and replaced by texts which indoctrinated the belief that a caste system is the only possible pattern on which an orderly society can be based. This propaganda was reinforced by genetic engineering – the insertion of the donkey's 'subservience' gene into human embryos – and the addition of chemicals to the water supply, intended to alter mental states and attitudes.

In the early years the plan was effected by weakening the population's curiosity, logical power, and questioning abilities through 'immunisations' universally administered, and by radically increasing the banality of television programmes and newspapers. As the population who had experienced relatively unfettered thought died off the manipulations were stepped up, so all new citizens could be physically and intellectually fitted from birth for their allotted roles ... This not only meant that people's intellectual powers were reduced and clouded, but also that the physiques of some were artificially restricted. The Elders' aim was to ensure the creation and perpetuation of their 'ideal state' through restraining the very existences of the human beings who constitute it.

It was necessary to interfere with the physical development of some children in order to suit them physically for the tasks they were to take on in 'adult' life. This meant that for some jobs, such as the non-automated inspection of pipelines, the cleaning of tower blocks and skyscrapers, and some types of mining, the physical development of some children was halted before puberty, and their intellectual development regulated according to the complexity of the task they were to perform. (If this seems incredible it is salutary to remember the not uncommon practice in India for desperate parents to cripple and mutilate their offspring in order to enable them to beg more successfully.) Many of Grand Thiam's children were intentionally prevented from fulfilling their natural physical and mental potentials in the interest of the society as a whole, as this interest was perceived by the Elders. In other words, these children were deliberately dwarfed ...

There is something intuitively disgraceful about the process of dwarfing.

Analysis of the theory and practice of health work shows that its underlying sense is the concern to remove or prevent obstacles to physical and mental growth. Health work strives to enable people to bring to fruition the range of potentials that lie latent within them. By educating, by curing disease, by mending broken bones, by developing personal power to conceive – to picture one's situation and future possibilities more clearly – health work is the antithesis of dwarfing.

Since it is an exact counter-balance to dwarfing (or 'the immoral') it follows that the health work endeavour is as objectively moral as it is possible to be. But because there are different types of health work, different senses of moral, and an indefinite range of contexts and ways in which health work can be carried out, it is not possible to say definitely that a particular intervention is *ideally* moral. It is also a mistake to assume that each attempt to create health will be as moral as any other ...[80]

Unfortunately, this argument was wishful thinking, taking several steps too far. Many societies do not, as a matter of fact, consider 'dwarfing' immoral. All they need do to oppose my heartfelt belief is to counter my intuition with a different intuition of their own. And after all, every western society produces 'cannon fodder' in one form or another – people whose use is mostly or even purely instrumental to the society in general (soldiers, factory workers, farm hands, taxi drivers and so on) – dispensable, disposable people whose identity does not matter one iota to the society as a whole.

As much as I wanted dwarfing to be the archetype of immorality I appreciate that it is possible to see dwarfing as immoral only within a framework of values and reasoning that considers it to be so (to be honest I knew this when I was writing *Ethics: The Heart of Health Care*). WITHIN the foundations theory of health[81] – the theory I was developing as I wrote the first edition of *Ethics: The Heart of Health Care* – dwarfing is indubitably immoral because according to the foundations theory the central point of working for health is to create autonomy – to enable people to achieve more than they could have done without your health intervention. Yet outside this special framework, dwarfing may or may not be immoral – it all depends on the particular moral framework from which actions are viewed.[74] For example, a framework that sees the basic point of life as the perpetuation of a particular national cause regardless of cost to individual human beings would not see the restriction of autonomy as a moral crime.

RELATIVISM HAS A POINT

Relativists undoubtedly have a point: if one person believes that everything that happens in the universe is God's will, while another sees a meaningless dance of electricity, then sooner or later they will have fundamentally different inter-pretations of events. Furthermore, anyone's judgement about the rightness and wrongness of values must depend upon an improvable value judgement, *ad infinitum*.

Nonetheless, it is one thing to accept that relativism has a certain plausibility, and quite another to say that this means we are all inescapably trapped in different bubbles of meaning. Certainly, the believer and the atheist will see some things differently, and will hold some incompatible views. But this does not mean they will have COMPLETELY relative outlooks. Nor does it mean they cannot experience, investigate and learn about an independent, external reality. And nor does it mean they cannot experience, investigate and learn about OTHER PEOPLE'S realities.

It is possible to understand relativism in a more constructive way. Indeed, this is an essential ingredient of the **VDM** project.

BEYOND-THE-EVIDENCE AND WITHIN-THE-EVIDENCE

In order to begin to understand the way past moral relativism, we must think a little more about the relationship between evidence and non-evidence.

EVIDENCE AND NON-EVIDENCE

By evidence I mean those matters of fact which exist whether we human beings like it or not. The evidence is those things which **just are** and which we cannot change.

For example, it **just is** the case that everything that is now alive will at some point be dead. It **just is** the case that if I shoot myself in the foot I will feel pain and I will bleed. It **just is** the case that an atomic bomb exploded at Hiroshima on Monday August 6th 1945. It **just is** the case that a large amount of energy can be released from a small amount of matter (expressed by the equation $E = mc^2$). And it **just is** the case that at this moment it is beautifully sunny outside and yet I am nevertheless sweating in my study trying to write this book.

The world is full of events, processes and natural laws that it makes no sense to doubt. However, as soon as we try to make SOCIAL sense of events and processes, **just is** certainty dissolves.

The place of evidence and non-evidence in our assessments of the world can be illustrated like this:

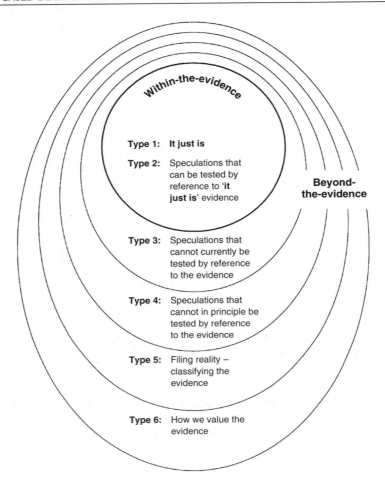

Figure 14   Types of evidence and non-evidence

The inner circle of this figure crudely depicts the world of evidence – the world that is what it is whatever we think of it. The ellipses outside the inner circle crudely depict different ways in which we interpret the inner circle evidence from a place beyond-the evidence. Here's a little more explanation:

WITHIN-THE-EVIDENCE

Type 1: The 'just is' realm

Many events and processes **just are**. With regard to breast cancer, it **just is** the case that:

> Breast cancer is the second leading cause of cancer death among North American women. Approximately 1 in 8.2 women will receive a diagnosis of breast cancer during her lifetime, and 1 in 30 will die of the disease.[82] Breast cancer incidence increases with

age,[82] and although significant progress has been made in identifying risk factors and genetic markers, more than 50 percent of cases occur in women without known major predictors.[83–87]

There is no doubting this evidence because it **just is** true, or at least it is as close to being true as statements which rely on human classifications can be. It is simply silly to believe that viewing this evidence from some non-scientific or non-medical conceptual scheme would alter the facts (the events and processes could undoubtedly be given different names and ascribed non-medical causes, but this would not alter the fact that the cancerous cells exist).

Type 2: Testable speculations

There are speculations that can be tested by reference to the **just is** evidence. The point of making such scientific speculations is to extend the **just is** realm as far as possible – to assess evidence, to combine it with other evidence, to apply research methods to see if the evidence really is **just is** – to get closer and closer to the empirical truth (even though science can never enter Plato's **Division One** – see p. 24 above). For example, the statements 'screening of women aged 40–49 by mammography can reduce the death rate from breast cancer'; 'life stress is a significant factor in the causation of breast cancer' are both testable.

BEYOND-THE-EVIDENCE

Type 3: Speculations that cannot currently be tested

The more we find that the evidence will not yield the explanations we require, the closer we move toward the realm beyond-the-evidence. We might call the first level beyond-the evidence **Type 3**.

Our speculations may be untestable:

(a) Because we do not yet have adequate techniques to do the tests (for example, we do not possess sophisticated enough methods properly to understand the depth and subtlety of human personality)

(b) Because reality is too complex for us to determine whether our speculations are correct (for example, the causes of breast cancer may be so wide, variable and unpredictable that we might never be able to establish a pattern beyond reasonable doubt, simply because the interplay between all the relevant factors defies human comprehension).

Type 4: Speculations that cannot in principle be tested

'It was pre-destined that Amy would experience breast cancer aged 43' and 'Amy's illness is the result of bad karma' are examples of this type, since both speculations are matters of faith.

Type 5: Human classifications – ways of filing reality

Type 5 is an important, pervasive and yet undernoticed feature of human life. Not only do we continually make instinctive and intentional beyond-the-evidence decisions to classify evidence into categories, we must do so if we are to make any sense of things at all.

We have to classify the world in order to think about it and act in it. For instance, unless we demarcate desirable behaviour from antisocial behaviour, normal thinking from abnormal thinking, and illness from non-illness – and make countless other daily distinctions – we are powerless to negotiate our social environment.

Many of our classifications stem directly from the evidence. For example, it **just is** the case that certain types of animal cannot reproduce with other types of animal. We have chosen to label these reproductive groups 'species', a decision which assists us in other speculations about biology and evolution.[88] It also **just is** the case that heavy bodies are attracted to the earth. We assume there must be an invisible force at work, which we call gravity – a classification that seems to help us understand some of the workings of the universe.[89] And of course we have created taxonomies of disease (infection by micro-organism, for example) that directly reflect the evidence as it **just is**.

The trouble is that we tend to believe that classifications (like sanity and insanity) that stem from beyond-the-evidence are just as certain as those (like sentient and non-sentient) that come from within it – they can seem to us to be just as factual as the laws of biology and physics. In western societies, for example, 'family' (meaning Mum, Dad, the children and a few close relatives) is commonly thought of as a unit of reality – something that just exists. And yet it is very obviously we who name different collections of individuals. We take the unadorned evidence of relationship (be it blood group, genetics, physical resemblance or merely geographical proximity) and label it 'family'. But this label does not exist outside human convention. As most people know, 'family' has different meanings in different cultures – for example, Maori consider family to be *whanau* or *iwi* (broader notions than the typical Western one).

'Intelligence' is conventionally defined as a capacity to understand verbal nuance, visual pattern and mathematical relationship. This classification has become so enshrined in western culture that entire careers can depend on how well one does in intelligence tests. However, there is no reason other than convention why artistic skill, poetic ability, the ability to empathise, or musical talent should not be considered the essence of intelligence. Educational philosophers, for example, define a variety of *intelligences* – linguistic, logical, musical, spatial, bodily, inter- and intra-personal, amongst others – challenging the assumption that intelligence is something that can be measured by a conventional IQ test.[90]

To make this quite clear: intelligence is not a **just is** unit of reality, intelligence is what we say it is. And the same is true of many other segments of the world we have chosen to categorise. It is even true of addiction:

> Since the eighteenth century, western man has organised particular behaviours into a specific, unitary phenomenon – namely, 'addiction' – as if this combination of behaviours is a distinct and real entity. The reasons why this combination of behaviours is created is not different from the reasons why the behavioural entity 'possessed by the devil' was created as the by-product of a past, religious, world view...'Addiction' is easily recognised by the culturally initiated, in the same way as in voodoo the impact of particular Spirits is

recognised out of behavioural elements that a non-initiated person would not even see, or would understand in a completely different way.[91]

Addiction exists as a category because we have taken some features of the **just is** world, seen them as significant, and lumped them together into a parcel that makes sense for us, at our time and in our culture. Of course some people develop habits and crave for one thing or another. But – like all the hundreds of other supposed mental illnesses – addiction exists as a category mainly because we want it to – it is an explanation that in some way fits with the evidence, and in some way suits us.

We are surrounded by an endless tangle of undefined processes, events and things – and we are driven to make sense of them: we seem to be irresistibly programmed to be the world's librarians. We file reality – as diseases, as illnesses, as measurements, as work, as leisure, as dates, as chunks of time, as charity, as right and wrong: we take the evidence, we decide its significance, we make it meaningful.

Type 6: How we value the evidence

Whether we realise it or not, we frequently interpret the evidence in accord with our moral preferences. And the way we value the evidence in turn affects and is affected by our speculations and classifications (see **Figure 19** below). For example, we may believe that human beings are entirely responsible for our actions (a **Type 4** speculation that cannot in principle be tested by reference to the evidence), that we should therefore be held accountable for these actions (a **Type 5** judgement that there is accountability and non-accountability and a **Type 6** judgement that it is good to hold people to account), and that we should be punished – as criminals – for unacceptable actions (a **Type 5** classification between criminals and non-criminals and a **Type 6** judgement that criminals ought to be punished). Or we may hold that sometimes people become mentally ill (a **Type 5** judgement) and – when we do become ill – that we should not be held responsible for our actions (judgements of **Type 5** and 6). All of these judgements about the evidence quite clearly arise from beyond it.

It is beyond doubt that evidence must be framed by human speculations, classifications, drives and instincts, social environment and history, and our personal preferences or values:

> . . . it is not possible to distinguish evidence about effectiveness and safety from values in a clear and mutually exclusive way . . . there are cultural differences in the way in which evidence is interpreted and decisions are made . . . people in the United States (are more willing) to intervene than decision-makers in Canada when presented with the same evidence.[92]

We are accustomed to thinking that our decisions take place mostly or entirely within-the-evidence, using Spock-reason. Yet the reality is that all our decision-making emanates from beyond-the-evidence.

Now it's easy to understand the breast cancer controversy described in **Chapter One** (p. 19 above).

MAMMOGRAPHY CONTROVERSY – SUMMARY

NIH Interpretation:

- Routine screening of 10,000 women aged 40 to 49 will lengthen the lives of approximately 0 to 10 of them
- To lengthen one life, approximately 2500 women will have to undergo regular screening

US Congress and the *New York Times* disagree with **NIH**:

- Accuse **NIH** of 'fraud' and 'condemning women to death'
- National Cancer Advisory Board (**NCAB**) reviews the **NIH** judgement
- **NCAB** – screening will decrease mortality by 17 per cent (saving hundreds of lives annually)
- **NCAB** Vote 17 for and 1 against: 1–2 year mammography for 40s women

Same Evidence – Different Values:

- **NIH** and **NCAB** had the same evidence but chose to select different aspects
- **NIH**:...of 10,000 women aged 40 to 49 screening will lengthen the lives of approximately 0 to 10 of them...=**NO!**
- **NCAB**:...screening will decrease mortality by 17 per cent (saving hundreds of lives annually)...=**YES!**

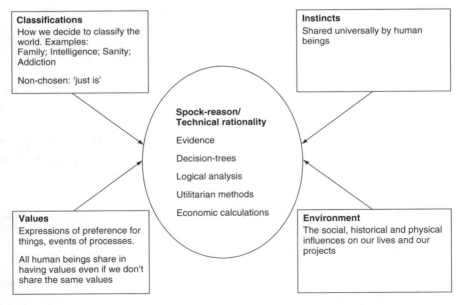

Figure 15 If you can't see the boxes you cannot understand the bubble – you need to know the frame to appreciate the picture

The reason the artist's friend could not see her shell picture was simply because he couldn't see its frame.

The evidence – the research papers, the medical histories, the fact that the incidence of breast cancer increases with age, the scientific calculations – is inside the Spock-bubble. Everything else – I am tempted to say everything that really matters – is on the outside. In order to understand why **NIH** and **NCAB** arrived at such conflicting recommendations, apparently on the basis of exactly the same evidence, it is necessary to try to understand the **classifications** the committee members used, their **instincts** (what were they frightened of? What did they hope for?), their **values** (what did they want to happen? How much did they desire the funding?) and their social and physical **environment** (what pressures were they under?).

Without a doubt, there were significantly different factors outside the Spock-bubble for the different committees. The reasons why we want to make decisions exist OUTSIDE the bubble – they form it and create its boundaries. When we forget this – when we are so caught up within our Spock-bubbles that we cannot see their boundaries and cannot see alternative bubbles either – we are in very deep trouble.

RATIONAL FIELDS

'Rational field' is a less engaging, more academic term for a Spock-bubble. Rational fields and their causative influences provide a means of working practically to improve the social world, using evidence and values in their proper balance.[93]

All rational fields have the same basic structure.[94–98] They are formed by any kind of problem-solving behaviour, and can therefore be any size from minuscule to enormous. A rational field is usually created either by an instinct or a value-judgement or both (a rational field can also be created by a social, physical or mental pressure). These instincts or judgements generate goals and sub-goals, strategies and sub-strategies, each of which maintain the rational field.

NATURAL AND MANUFACTURED RATIONAL FIELDS

NATURAL RATIONAL FIELDS

It **just is** the case that the living world is composed of innumerable rational fields (though they are often described by different names). A plant striving to grow and to propagate is a rational field. A bacterium is a rational field, a cell in a body is a rational field, a gene is a rational field, organs in the human body are rational fields, a developing person is a rational field: anything instinctively purposive is a natural rational field. All the above examples have goals and sub-goals, strategies and sub-strategies, each of which maintain their respective rational fields. If new problems emerge, each rational field may expand or adapt in order to try to deal with them. For example, in ideal circumstances a plant will grow and produce many seeds. If there is a drought, or if the plant is attacked by insects, or if there is excessive wind, then if it can it will adapt its goals and strategies accordingly (perhaps it will make only one fruit instead of many, or perhaps it will produce special chemicals to repel further insect attack, or perhaps it will grow extra roots as an anchor). This adaptive behaviour is true of any natural, goal-directed system.[98]

This **just is** the way the world is – natural rational fields exist within-the-evidence.

No natural rational field is wholly independent – because of the world's interconnectedness – but any rational field must have at least one distinct purpose and strategy by which to pursue it.

The point of rational fields is the exercise of autonomy, and the point of associated rational fields is to provide the wherewithal for autonomy while being autonomous themselves.

MANUFACTURED RATIONAL FIELDS

Manufactured rational fields are different from natural ones. They are also goal-directed (they must be to be rational fields) but they tend to be more erratic and unstable than natural rational fields, since they are formed by human beyond-the-evidence assumptions and decisions.

Natural rational fields are all around and within us. Manufactured rational fields are formed and sustained by our classifications of reality (**Type 5**), our values (**Type 6**), and our instincts (see **Figure 15** above). Manufactured rational fields can be as small as a plan to read a book with a glass of wine this evening, and as big as it is possible for any human institution to be. Conventional health services are manufactured rational fields, Microsoft is a manufactured rational field, Microsoft's marketing department is a manufactured rational field, and so is psychiatry, nursing, a badminton club, and the law of the land – every system designed by humans to achieve a purpose is a manufactured rational field.

Once we can properly recognise manufactured rational fields for what they are we can take control over them. Once we know what we are dealing with we do not have to fall into rational fields that suit other people more than they suit us, and we do not have to follow particular goal-directed paths in the false belief that these paths are all there is.

An example of a simple manufactured rational field

A traveller unexpectedly lost in a foreign city, unable to speak or read the native language, must define a goal and devise ways to achieve it if she wants to regain her bearings. She might think: I don't want to be lost (a value judgement or instinct which defines the Spock-bubble's perimeter), if I find the central railway station I will probably find a map (two related goals), if I draw a picture of a train with a question mark and show it around I may get directions to the station (two related strategies), first I need to find some paper (sub-goal)...and so on. By doing these things she creates a small rational field. As she formulates and tries strategies to achieve her goal the field expands. As soon as she is successful, the rational field dissipates.

An example of a complex manufactured rational field

Large organisations such as hospitals and commercial companies create and perpetuate vast and complex rational fields. Just like the traveller's field, these larger fields are initially created by classifications and value-judgements or instincts (we must treat disease, we must improve our brand recognition) which generate further goals and sub-goals, strategies and sub-strategies, each of which contributes to the rational field's evolution.

To describe the relationships between the goals, strategies and means of an organisation the size of **BP** is a virtually impossible task – even the most determinedly extensive depiction of **BP**'s rational field would be an oversimplification (and would be at least as silly as the silliest extension of Spock-reason). Fortunately the exact details don't matter for present purposes. Rather it is the basic *structure* and *formation* of rational fields that needs to be understood. If you know this then you can assess any manufactured rational field for coherence and value, and can also manufacture a rational field according to your own classifications and values.

THE RATIONAL FIELD TEMPLATE

All rational fields, whether natural or manufactured, can be very crudely depicted as in **Figure 16**.

A plant's instinctive rational field response to an attack by an insect might be illustrated by **Figure 17**. **Figure 17** is a natural rational field. Its means are well-related to its goals, and its goals are compatible. Some loss of optimal normal functioning is tolerated in order to achieve **Goal Z**.

Microsoft's manufactured rational field response to the surprise emergence of revolutionary software from a rival company might (again very crudely) be illustrated as in **Figure 18**. In **Figure 18** the company's decision is to adopt Strategy Two, to try to prevent the rival launching its product in order to give Microsoft time to increase its own research and development efforts. It is very easy to see how decision trees and other cost-benefit based assessments might be built into the rational field.

It is not suggested that the solution offered in **Figure 18** is what Microsoft would actually do. Rather, it is an illustrative response, meant only to introduce the idea of a manufactured rational field.

At this stage, the main points to note about rational fields are:

1. That even simply expressed, the rational field template is useful because it enables decision-makers to state their most important goals, crudely to check whether these goals are compatible with each other, to define and lay out different strategies, to see how these impact on the goals (some may fit with one goal but not another, for example), to state the primary means for achieving any goals, and to assess whether the means, strategies and goals are coherent and efficient (standard technical rationality in other words).

2. Even more important, it is possible, by using the rational field template, to see how a rational field is formed from beyond-the-evidence. In addition to a simple internal field made up of means, strategies and goals, the rational field template shows four boxes – one for instincts, one for classifications, one for values, and one for environment – that explain why the internal goals and strategies have been selected. Instincts, classifications, values and the environment shape the rational field – they form its walls. Usually, in our social affairs, we tend not to notice or we play down these elements. But they are crucial for the rational field template. Only by properly understanding them can we understand our rational fields, and judge between them comprehensively.

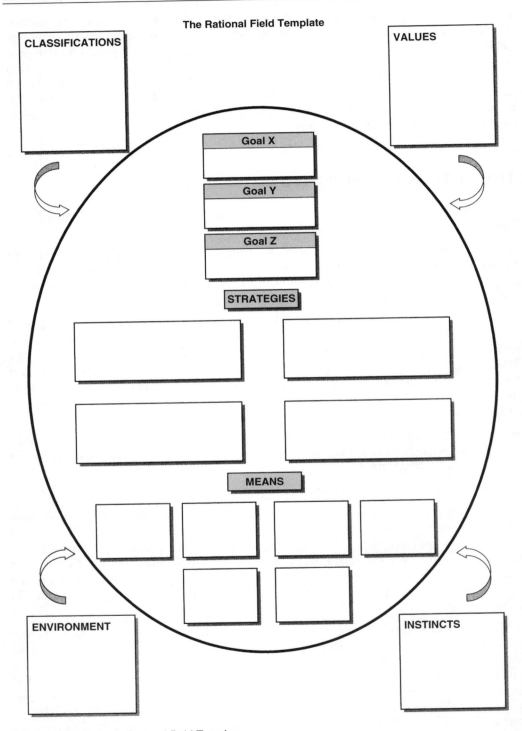

Figure 16   The Basic Rational Field Template

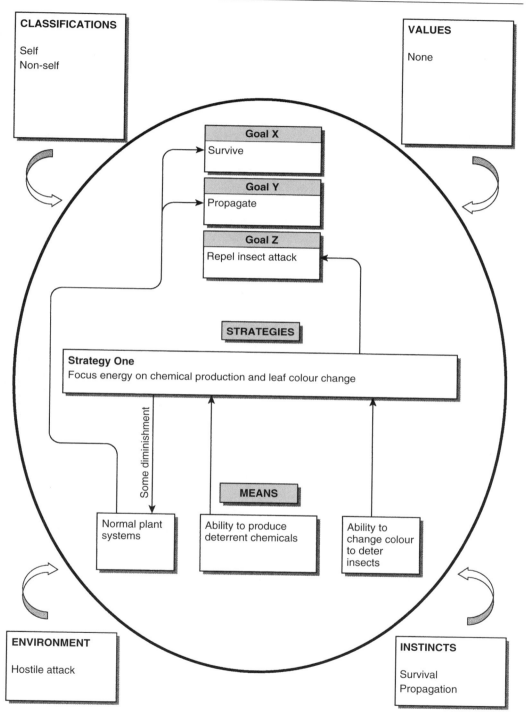

Figure 17   The Rational Field Template simply expressed for a plant's reponse to insect attack (this is a natural rational field)

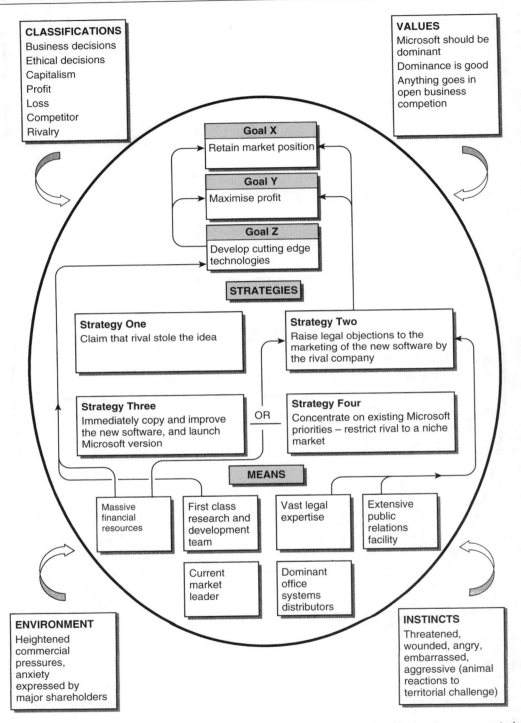

CLASSIFICATIONS
Business decisions
Ethical decisions
Capitalism
Profit
Loss
Competitor
Rivalry

VALUES
Microsoft should be
dominant
Dominance is good
Anything goes in
open business
competion

Goal X
Retain market position

Goal Y
Maximise profit

Goal Z
Develop cutting edge
technologies

STRATEGIES

Strategy One
Claim that rival stole the idea

Strategy Two
Raise legal objections to the
marketing of the new software by
the rival company

Strategy Three
Immediately copy and improve
the new software, and launch
Microsoft version

OR

Strategy Four
Concentrate on existing Microsoft
priorities – restrict rival to a niche
market

MEANS

Massive
financial
resources

First class
research and
development
team

Vast legal
expertise

Extensive
public
relations
facility

Current
market
leader

Dominant
office
systems
distributors

ENVIRONMENT
Heightened
commercial
pressures,
anxiety
expressed by
major shareholders

INSTINCTS
Threatened,
wounded, angry,
embarrassed,
aggressive (animal
reactions to
territorial challenge)

Figure 18 The Rational Field Template crudely expressed for Microsoft's response to a rival
company's revolutionary software (this is a manufactured rational field)

Filling in the instinct, value, classification and environment boxes can be an uncomfortable process, particularly for people who have never conceived that their world is an option rather than a necessary reality. To have these very basic human judgements forced into the open can feel like a home invasion (which it is, in a way). But it is necessary if we are to be able to explore our thinking and our policies open-mindedly.

Evidence is never ultimately decisive when human beings make decisions. Trace any decision back to its roots and you will, without exception, find a value of some kind. It might, for example, be decided that 'we' (i.e. law abiding, non-terrorist citizens) obviously need better security procedures at international airports – given the overwhelming recent evidence of organised violence (I write this in November 2004). Yet this is not an obvious decision but a judgement based on values (such as our very understandable preference to feel as secure as possible inside airports), human classification (there are 'terrorists' and there are 'the rest of us') and instinct (most people are naturally afraid of hidden threats).

We are unlikely to change our preference for safety, and our instincts **just are**. However, it is open to us to alter our classification of others (for example, from 'terrorists' to 'neighbours') and to do so on the ground of an alternative value – perhaps the Christian edict that we should love our neighbours as ourselves. If we were to start from this latter value base we would come up with a very different strategy from one derived from the atavistic snarl that we should 'take revenge on evil terrorists everywhere'.

Once we have decided we need better security at international airports, subsidiary questions follow – for example, 'How shall we meet our perceived need?' These questions also require values if they are to be answered. Shall we, for instance, work out what sort of security to provide according to cost, aesthetics, or civil liberties? Shall we invest more on armed police or more on improved surveillance technology? Shall we make a truce with our enemies? Or shall we simply decide according to 'what works best'? (But of course, there is no escape: 'what works best' depends on what is meant by 'best', and what counts as 'best' depends on human preferences. Value judgements are everywhere.)

THE RELATIONSHIP BETWEEN CLASSIFICATIONS, VALUES, INSTINCTS AND ENVIRONMENT

It is worth noting that since definitions of classification, value, instinct and environment are themselves subject to interpretation there is room for speculation about their place and relationship. For example, one might ask, are instincts values or are they the source of values?

One might argue this either way:

(a) Instincts are values: it is my instinct to avoid large objects speeding toward me. My instinct exists to prevent injury or death as a result of a collision. Thus one might say that my instinct is a value, because it is an inherent preference toward life and safety rather than death or injury.
(b) Instincts are the source of values: taking the same example, one might also argue that my instinct to avoid injury and death is the root of my valuing life and safety (the instinct is not a value but an inbuilt and unexamined aspect of me).

One can imagine arguments claiming that a value can override an instinct – for example, if I value my child's safety more than my own I might deliberately place myself in danger to save her, overcoming my instinct for self-preservation and implying that values are more fundamental than instincts. The alternative argument, of course, is that my instinct to save my child is the source of my preference to put myself in danger rather than her.

I cannot imagine that this matters too much either way, but it may be salutary to acknowledge the potential complexity.

It could also be argued that there is a two-way arrow between values and classifications – that our values cause us to create our classifications of the world beyond the 'just is' realm, and that in turn our classifications affect our values. It might also be claimed that our social, psychological and physical environments create at least some of our values and instincts, and so on.

The relationship between these factors might look something like **Figure 19**, in a very simplified form. One might also invent a scheme that asserts a hierarchy of values. Perhaps like this:

Lower preferences/values

These might be basic preferences such as: I like food, I like sex, I like this mood-altering substance, I like the after-effects of exercise, I like this picture, I like this object, I like this sensation and so on.

Higher preferences/values

These might be reasoned preferences: intellectual pleasures; valuing literature and music; long-term commitment to relationships; deeply reasoned, argued preferences for social projects, and so on.

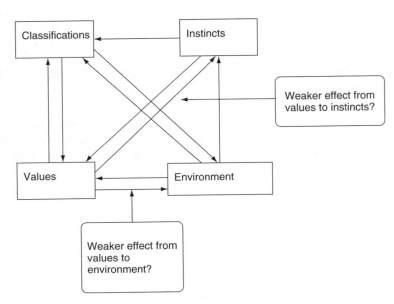

Figure 19   A possible relationship between values, classifications, instincts and environment

But such distinctions are merely the stuff of arid academic debate. What really matters is that the values which lie behind practical decision-making are revealed – in order that we can see how they influence things. If some decision-makers assume a different hierarchy from other decision-makers this may be intellectually interesting, but it is much more important that we get their different classifications, instincts, values and environments transparent and on the table – so that we can try to establish how one source leads to a different Spock-bubble from another source.

THE TRUTH ABOUT RELATIVISM

We are now in a much better position to understand how different people and different groups of people come to see the world so differently from one another.

TAKING A STEP BACK TO TRANSCEND RELATIVISM

We continually create billions of natural and manufactured rational fields of varying degrees of compatibility and incompatibility. But we do not have to be trapped within specific rational fields. So long as we are aware of the processes which generate any given field we can rise above it to consider (perhaps even to establish) what created it. We KNOW that manufactured rational fields don't just emerge out of thin air, but are caused by a complex combination of instincts, values, classifications and environments. Our challenge, whenever we want to understand Spock-bubbles in context, is to investigate these causes and review the merits of the Spock-bubble/rational field in the light of our investigation.

If we take just the basic **Figure 15** above it may look as if we are trapped. It may seem that we are corralled into particular Spock-bubbles – inevitably forced into restricted rational fields by the surrounding causes (just as psychiatrists, soldiers, politicians and lawyers are forced more and more to inhabit specific technical fields – buying into their classifications and values in order to be allowed to BE psychiatrists or soldiers at all).

But **Figure 15** is merely an illustrative figure. To see the real picture you need to imagine billions of mini-rational fields (the ellipses), each with its surrounding causes (the boxes) as shown in **Figure 20**.

At any time any human being will have innumerable rational fields in existence (I need to finish this section by 12.15 p.m. in order to go swimming, I need to lower the volume of my rock music so I can think clearly, I need to drink my cup of tea, I need to stretch my arms, I need to think about rationality, my body is breathing, I am perspiring, my heart is beating, haemoglobin is pumping around my body, I can hear birds singing in the bush outside etc. etc. etc., almost *ad infinitum*...).

It is quite obvious that each of us can transcend our OWN rational fields to see them simultaneously, and quite often we can clearly understand their causes. Think about your own rational fields/Spock-bubbles right now. As you do so you create yet another rational field (one with the goal of reviewing your current rational fields and their causes, created by your understanding the classification 'rational field' and your valuing giving my argument a reasonable hearing). This additional rational field

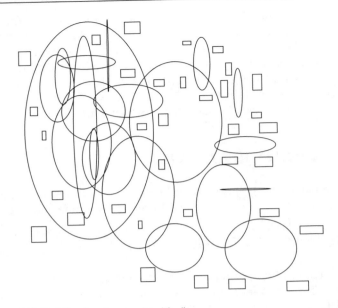

Figure 20   Rational field reality (vastly oversimplified)

gives us a mind's eye view of the sea of rational fields which constitute ourselves and our projects.

We never have to be trapped within any manufactured rational field, so long as we can take this step back. We can even see this mind's eye rational field as we think about it, so creating a further rational field (**Figure 22**), and so on.

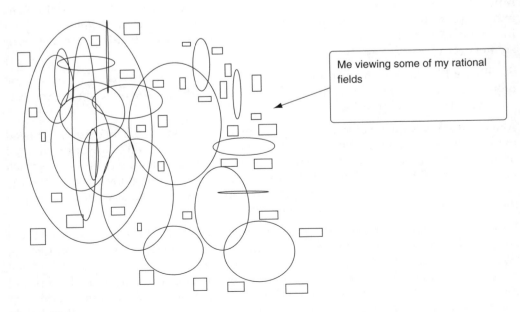

Me viewing some of my rational fields

Figure 21

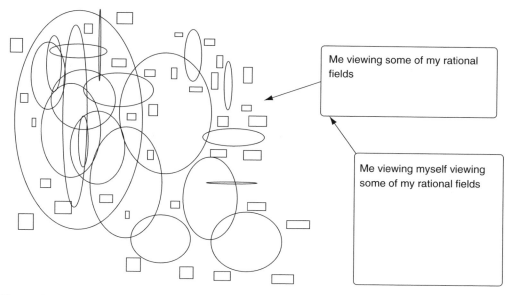

Figure 22

We can sensibly extend this to include ourselves viewing rational fields that are not our own – see **Figures 23** and **24**.

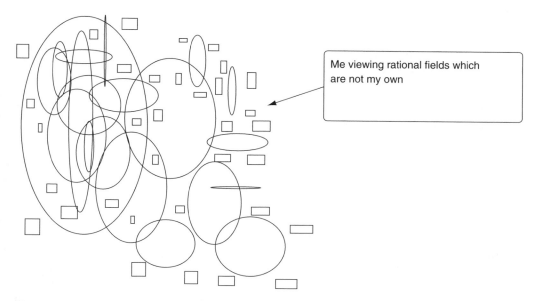

Figure 23

and so on:

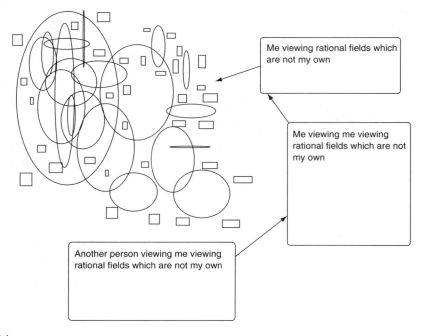

Figure 24

and so on.

From an academic point of view this may look absurd – an infinite regress (like oneself thinking about oneself thinking about oneself thinking about oneself thinking...). But in reality this **just is** what happens (in reality I just can't think about myself thinking about myself thinking *ad infinitum*).

In a way, it would make sense to call the Spock-bubble AND its surrounding influences 'a rational field', since this would properly extend our understanding of rationality (rationality is essentially a successful balance of logic and emotion). However, it makes practical sense to retain the present configuration, which labels Spock-rationality alone 'the rational field', so we shall stick with this label.

WHAT THIS MEANS

What all this means is that we can try to understand Kate and Lucy's rational fields and their causes, and we can also judge between them and understand why we judge between them (see **Chapter Two**, pp. 42–44). Because I can compare Kate and Lucy's rational fields to my own preferred rational field for Terry and her mother I am helped to see a range of possibility – or at the very least to resist arrogance (I can certainly see that my own rational field is informed by a theory of health in addition to the four factors drawn in **Figure 15**).[99] I find that I prefer Lucy's rational field with regard to diagnosing and helping Terry because my values and instincts tend toward seeing people as suffering beings struggling to find a way forward, rather than clinical pathologies.

This does not mean I can say that Kate is morally wrong, or that objectively Lucy's rational field is to be preferred over Kate's. But it does mean that I can say why I have my preference, in a clear and detailed way. It also means that I can stand back from my judgement between the two rational fields to take a mind's eye view of myself making this judgement – in other words I can view the rational field of myself making this decision. I can't view this Spock-bubble dispassionately – you can't be a human being without constant passion – but I can see it and I can assess it for its causes: preference, classification, instinct, environment, and its logic. This reviewing may even give me cause to change my mind.

Somehow we have to distance ourselves – even if only a little. We can all become philosophers, critics, examiners of as much as is open to us to examine with the intellects and emotions we have.

Perpetual reflection and reviewing, appreciating the proper balance between reason and passion is a far more optimistic standpoint than[100] accepting absolute relativism. It raises the prospect of knowledge, understanding and conversation and is exactly the intent of the **VDM** systems explained in the final chapters.

Trying to understand the interplay between rational fields is something every one of us can attempt. Everyone – Muslim or Christian, man or woman, black or white, Vulcan or human – can understand the concept of rational fields and every competent person has a grasp of logic and reason at some level. We share in this understanding because we are human beings – and this is the great hope for us. See values in their proper relationship with logic and there is real hope for honesty, openness and insight (though never full agreement) rather than covertness, hostility and blindness to other people's points of view.

By standing back I can review my classifications, instincts, values, environment and logic whenever I want to. I have the potential to decide if the rational field I am currently using is TRULY the rational field I want to be using. Isn't this what we should all be doing? See **Figure 25**.

If I am right about rational fields, the world is a great mass of bubbles – billions and trillions of bubbles – bubbles everywhere, each of which is a rational field, overlapping in ways that cannot be pictured by us.

The big picture is like a many-dimensional snowstorm. We would need to be able to think in other dimensions to see rational fields properly. Whereas snowflakes exist in discreet places, rational fields can be in many places at once, and can overlap in multiple ways with multiple other rational fields, in an incredible complexity. For example, one person's rational field to go to a memorial service is not separate from others within him (his memories, his fears, his hopes, his sense of self). It connects to his other rational fields and other people's rational fields in all sorts of ways – so the whole picture cannot be seen at once – it can be depicted only if we artificially abstract individuals and fields from the great overall mass.

As far as this idea can be explained, rational fields constantly overlap, merge, collide, burst, pop into existence and pop out of existence – in a sub-atomic world of overwhelming complexity.

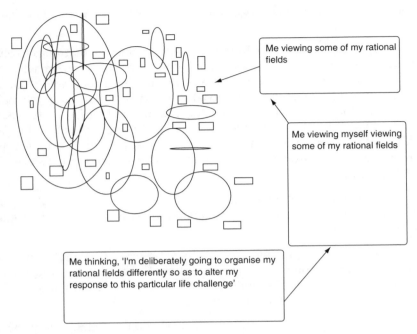

Me viewing some of my rational fields

Me viewing myself viewing some of my rational fields

Me thinking, 'I'm deliberately going to organise my rational fields differently so as to alter my response to this particular life challenge'

Figure 25   Using the mind's eye to reflect on and consider changing the rational fields which one can change

RATIONAL FIELD PHILOSOPHY REVEALS THE FOLLY OF POST-MODERNISM

As far as I can understand the post-modernist position about 'all truth being relative' – and I confess that my understanding is rather limited – it seems to be something like this: the basic assumptions about science, reality, morality or anything else that societies take for granted as truths are entirely dependent upon power. Power is primarily wielded by the use of language in 'discourses'. These discourses are self-contained worlds of meaning – their meaning comes only from the internal uses of language and not from the external world (they are pseudo Spock-bubbles, with meaning inside them rather than causing them). Everybody 'inhabits' a number of discourses, for example, I may be said to belong to the 'homeschooling' discourse (because my wife and I homeschool our children), the 'white middle class middle-aged male discourse' (obviously ☺) and the 'ex-patriot discourse' because I live 12,000 miles away from the country in which I was born.

The idea seems to be that discourses come into being as dominant groups of people assert the interpretations of the world they favour. These dominant groups allow only those ways of seeing the world that suit them – so, for example, groups of indigenous people may decide that everyone should support the cultural values of minority cultures and so invent the notion 'cultural safety'. If they are powerful enough they can create a discourse about race relations that allows no term other than 'cultural safety' – effectively limiting the available meanings within the 'race relations discourse' to the one meaning they want. The US news media's use of the word 'terrorist' as if 'terrorist' is a factual term is another example. According to the disciples of Michael

Foucault, this has the effect of preventing most people even conceiving that Osama Bin Laden might not be a terrorist as a matter of fact. Equally, the powerful supporters of Osama Bin Laden allow only the expression 'freedom fighter' to apply to him, so preventing people within their discourse imagining him as anything other than a freedom fighter.

So, a discourse can be thought of as:

> ... an instutionalized way of thinking, a social boundary defining what can be said about a specific topic. Discourses are (said) to affect our views on all things ... it is not possible to escape discourse.[101]

If this extreme relativist view is true then we are all confined within limited worlds of meaning created by the human struggle for power, trapped within impenetrable bubbles like No. 6 in the classic 60s series, *The Prisoner*.[102] Without discourse to provide meaning we are like a newborn baby without social language – we cannot understand anything since all understanding of the world must come from within discourse. What's more, since power changes hands from time to time we are constantly at the mercy of changes in discourse. If the discourse has moved on, or has been moved on, what we were able to think yesterday may not be thinkable today.

George Orwell may have had something like this in mind when he described Winston's job at the Ministry of Truth, where he was employed to rewrite history and progressively reduce the number of words available in public dictionaries.

Significantly, however, even though Winston was subject to extensive brainwashing, for most of the novel he retains his scepticism, spirit and logic; capacities which cause him to write in his diary:

> I understand how: I do not understand why.[103]

At the time he wrote this Winston didn't understand why anyone would want to rewrite history because he was not privy to the dominant discourse. He couldn't see the world as the Party saw the world.

(Ironically, in the case of **discourse relativism**, the reverse applies as far as I'm concerned. I can just about understand why someone might want to advance such a view yet I am quite unable to understand how it is supposed to work.)

We'll leave it to O'Brien, Winston's torturer, to explain why the Party wants power. He speaks to Winston in the torture room:

> 'And now let us get back to the question of "how" and "why". You understand well enough how the Party maintains itself in power. Now tell me why we cling to power. What is our motive? Why should we want power?'[103]

> '... I will tell you the answer to my question. It is this. The Party seeks power entirely for its own sake. We are not interested in the good of others; we are interested solely in power. Not wealth or luxury or long life or happiness: only power, pure power ... The German Nazis and the Russian Communists came very close to us in their methods, but they never had the courage to recognize their own motives. They pretended, perhaps they even believed, that they had seized power unwillingly and for a limited time, and that just round the corner there lay a paradise where human beings would be free and equal. We are not like that. We know that no one ever seizes power with the intention of relinquishing it. Power is not a means, it is an end ... The object of persecution is persecution. The object of torture is torture. The object of power is power. Now do you begin to understand me?' (Chapter Three)[103]

The means of achieving this absolute power is very close to what it must be like to be overwhelmed by a discourse:

> 'Has it ever occurred to you that . . . [s]lavery is freedom . . . if [a human being] can make complete, utter submission, if he can escape from his identity, if he can merge himself in the Party so that he is the Party, then he is all-powerful and immortal. The second thing for you to realize is that power is power over human beings. Over the body but, above all, over the mind. Power over matter – external reality, as you would call it – is not important.'[103]

The Party wants everyone to think as they do because that will be the end of history – if they triumph there will be only one discourse left, and with everyone locked inside it there would be no chance of it ever changing. In order to inculcate Winston into the Party's discourse, the Party tortures him physically but they know that to succeed they must force him to relinquish his own discourse – only if he does that will he be ready to accept theirs.

The Party eventually succeeds in cruelly compelling Winston to realise that he left his old discourse behind and joined theirs when he denounced his love for Julia, his lover. This is poignantly confirmed in the final chapter in which Winston meets Julia by chance. They admit they each betrayed the other in the face of O'Brien's threats. Julia tells Winston that when the only way to save yourself from something you cannot endure is to make another person suffer instead, then you will readily agree to that suffering. No matter how much you pretend afterwards that you only did it to escape, you cannot escape the knowledge that at the crucial moment you willed the other person to suffer so you didn't have to.

> 'And then you say, "Don't do it to me, do it to somebody else, do it to So-and-so." And perhaps you might pretend, afterwards, that it was only a trick and that you just said it to make them stop and didn't really mean it. But that isn't true. At the time when it happens you do mean it. You think there's no other way of saving yourself, and you're quite ready to save yourself that way. You want it to happen to the other person. You don't give a damn what they suffer. All you care about is yourself.' (Final chapter)[103]

Winston could see the truth of this. After you'd betrayed them so willingly, he knew you could never feel the same way about the person you had betrayed.[104]

Finally Winston is absorbed into the Party's discourse:

> The trumpet-call had let loose an enormous volume of noise. Already an excited voice was gabbling from the telescreen, but even as it started it was almost drowned by a roar of cheering from outside. The news had run round the streets like magic. He could hear just enough of what was issuing from the telescreen to realize that it had all happened, as he had foreseen; a vast seaborne armada had secretly assembled a sudden blow in the enemy's rear, the white arrow tearing across the tail of the black. Fragments of triumphant phrases pushed themselves through the din: 'Vast strategic manoeuvre – perfect co-ordination – utter rout – half a million prisoners – complete demoralization – control of the whole of Africa – bring the war within measurable distance of its end victory – greatest victory in human history – victory, victory, victory!'

> Under the table Winston's feet made convulsive movements. He had not stirred from his seat, but in his mind he was running, swiftly running, he was with the crowds outside, cheering himself deaf. He looked up again at the portrait of Big Brother. The colossus that bestrode the world! . . . He loved Big Brother. (Final chapter)[103]

Presumably a post-modernist would say that at this point the discourse had finally gobbled Winston up completely.

HOW IS DISCOURSE RELATIVISM (OR ANY OTHER FORM) SUPPOSED TO WORK?

But do discourses really do this to us? Do they really so disable us that we can't think any other way than according to their rules? The trouble with relativism (of any sort) is that it is too simplistic, and seems wilfully to ignore the reality of the human condition. As we saw above (p. 51):

> ...different schemes of classification incorporate witches and tree spirits, phlogiston and the ether, electrons and magnetic fields....Schemes of concepts provide grids on which to base belief...[70]

> ...what is true for the Hopi is not so for us; what is true for Aristotle is not true for Galileo...[71]

and

> ...what counts as a good reason may be context-dependent. Galileo consulted observation and experiment, Bellarmine the scriptures; Evans-Pritchard the available evidence of causal connections, Azande the poison oracle. Each is equally enmeshed in a web of reasons, properly woven by its own standards from within but finally incapable of support from without.[72]

The implication of this is that discourses are all-encompassing – either you are in or you are out. If you believe in tree spirits you can't believe in magnetic fields, if you are from the Hopi tribe you will not understand *Coronation Street*.

Relativists have to paint a picture of large, incompatible discourses – relative cultures – or else face a *reductio ad absurdam* in which there is an infinite number of smaller and smaller discourses, leading ultimately to a desperate solipsism where everyone inhabits a personal discourse with no access to an external reality and no way to be sure their personal set of meanings is shared by anyone else.

But both of these – the big discourses and the infinitesimally small ones – are fictions dreamt up by academics who apparently have nothing better to do. They may 'work' in abstract texts but they take little or no account of what life is actually like. All you need to do to see this is to see the world as it is – with billions upon billions of rational fields, natural and manufactured, big and small, long- and short-lived, apart and overlapping in great complexity – a colossal dance of meaningful bubbles of thought and action. See the world like this and the idea that we are trapped in unfathomable 'discourses' evaporates instantly.

It may not be possible to love Big Brother AND to love selflessly, but it is clearly possible to believe in witchcraft and electrons (Arthur Koestler[105] and Colin Wilson do[106]), scriptures and empirical observation (the Catholic church does[107]), and to understand that both Aristotle and Galileo were scientists with a lot more in common than not.

Consider this newspaper report:

Sunday November 21, 2004
The Observer

The girl's white shirt was clogged with blood. Her attacker had broken down the bathroom door to get to her – the floor was slippery with her blood. He'd set about her with such ferocity that the tip of the kitchen knife had broken off, stabbing her 11 times and then slitting her throat. She was 16, and he was her father.

Abdulla Yones killed his daughter Heshu in their flat on the third floor of Charles Hocking House, a dismal council block in Acton, west London. Two days earlier, he had received an anonymous letter at the south London offices of the Kurdish PUK, where he worked as a volunteer, disclosing that it was known in the community that she had a boyfriend, and claiming that she was behaving like a prostitute. After Abdulla Yones was sentenced to life imprisonment, he said he'd been forced to kill Heshu because he'd been placed in an untenable position.

In Yones's mind, there was a stain on his family. It is difficult to understand what exactly about Heshu's fairly typical teenage behaviour was at fault here – liking make-up? Having a boyfriend? The boyfriend not being entirely welcome to the family? – but perhaps the offence was less specific: Heshu wanted to assert her independence and, evidently, she was succeeding. Her father could not control her, and this was so shaming that it could only be overcome by her complete subjugation, by her death.

Honour killings often provoke smug responses from Westerners. The judge in Yones's murder trial concluded the case was 'in any view a tragic story of irreconcilable cultural differences between traditional Kurdish values and the values of Western society'. There is more than a whiff of cultural superiority here – but this is the same Western society that sees two women in Britain murdered by their partners every week.[108]

As distressing as this murder is, it is by no means impossible to understand it.

In summary, if you see the world as composed of rational fields – each created by at least one **instinct**, **classification**, **value** or **environmental** factor (usually many) – then you can stand back from the fields you are interested in:

- To see how they work logically (to study the technical rationality within the Spock-bubble)
- To see how their logic fits with other rational fields
- To see how they have been created
- To see how their classifications, instincts, values and environments compare with other fields' classifications, instincts, values and environments

And you can:

- Reject rational fields
- Choose one rational field over another
- Understand why you used to create rational fields you no longer create[109]
- Understand why your current rational fields may be better (or worse) than your old ones
- Gain insight – as you see how other people's apparently bizarre or irrational logic is created you can begin to see things as they do – but you don't need to relinquish your own preferred or instinctive rational fields in order to do this. In anything other than the extreme case endured by Winston it is possible to try to see the point of rational fields you have initially rejected – if this were impossible (and if we could not access the external world to test out our ideas) then we really would all be trapped forever in some all-pervading and impenetrable fog of meaning.

But we are not. We love. We fear. We aspire. We desire. We laugh. We cry. We play. We research. We learn. We grow. We can understand other people because they are like us, and we can understand apparently alien ideas so long as we know enough about their Spock-bubbles and the causes of their Spock-bubbles. We are human beings and therefore have to interpret the world as human beings – but we have ways of standing outside our prejudices. Perhaps we can never access eternal truths (whatever these may be) but we can sometimes reach outside ourselves, and we can sometimes change what we know and how we think.

SOME IMPLICATIONS OF USING RATIONAL FIELD PHILOSOPHY TO INFORM PRACTICAL DECISION-MAKING

The single most important consequence of values-based philosophy is the recognition that by using the notion of rational fields, every decision can be seen in a properly balanced perspective. Once the basic idea of rational fields is accepted, every decision can be seen as some combination of logic, evidence, convention, instinct and prefer-ence, and not merely a purely technical solution to some neutral problem arisen out of nowhere.

Once this insight is appreciated, the following situations are open to balanced analysis:

1. **A situation where two different rational fields A and B co-exist and where one is privileged for some reason (for example, by power, authority, or scientific status)**

If we can DISPLAY the whole fields AND their sources (i.e. if BOTH – including the privileged one, can be seen to emanate from values, instincts and classifications) then we can, by standing back, begin to make better informed decisions about which rational field to prefer. If in the end we retain the privileged field, we will do so with increased humility having better appreciated the structure of the alternative field, and its non-logical foundations.

For example:

The 'boxing champion'

Peter Breggin believes 'many of the symptoms associated with so-called schizophrenia are blatant attempts to compensate for humiliations experienced while growing up'. His understanding of mental illness may translated, without residue, into rational fields.

Breggin writes:

> I'm reminded of the fifteen-year-old frail, frightened boy who came into the hospital declaring that he was a boxing champion. He even could describe his main bouts. His true story was one of being physically abused at home and dominated by bigger boys at school. With regularity, therapists see young men who attempt to bolster their self-esteem by declaring they are somebody extraordinarily important, when deep down they feel humiliated and worthless.[110]

Of course, the frail fifteen year old could conceivably be suffering from a brain abnormality that causes grandiose ideas. However, it is at least as conceivable – and infinitely more meaningful – that his rational field and his environment's rational field are so much at odds that something has to give, and of course the boy is infinitely less powerful than his environment. To over-simplify grossly, the situation might be characterised by **Figures 26** and **27**.

Looked at one way this is nothing more than a paraphrase of Breggin's account of the situ-ation. However, expressing things in this simple format allows a judgement about which (if any) rational field is a problem, allows the assessment of different rational fields, and suggests solutions that involve changing one or more rational fields – and not automatic-ally or necessarily the boy's.

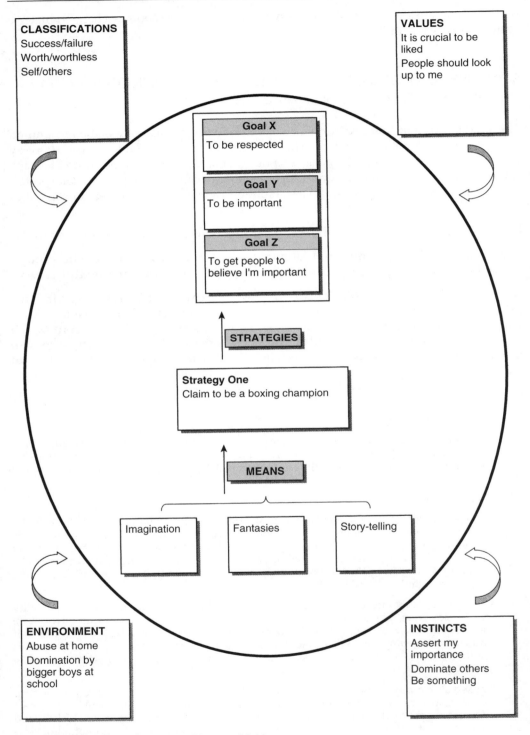

Figure 26   The 'Boxing Champion's' rational field

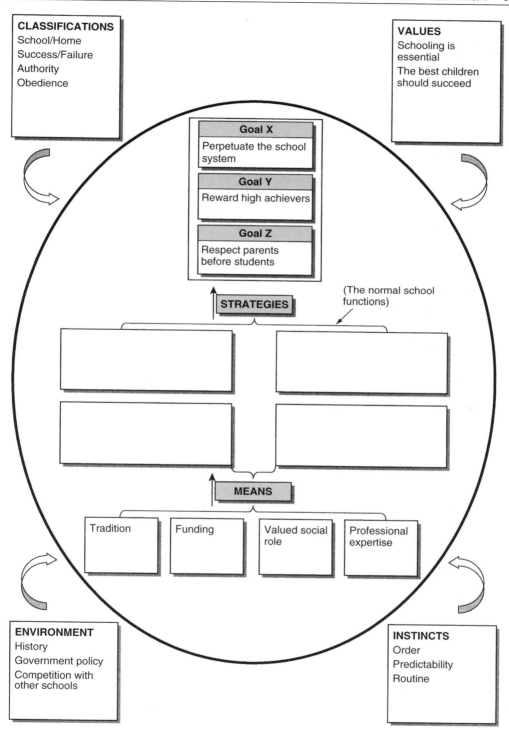

CLASSIFICATIONS
School/Home
Success/Failure
Authority
Obedience

VALUES
Schooling is
essential
The best children
should succeed

Goal X
Perpetuate the school
system

Goal Y
Reward high achievers

Goal Z
Respect parents
before students

(The normal school
functions)

STRATEGIES

MEANS

| Tradition | Funding | Valued social role | Professional expertise |

ENVIRONMENT
History
Government policy
Competition with
other schools

INSTINCTS
Order
Predictability
Routine

Figure 27   The 'Boxing Champion's' school's prevailing rational field

For one example, a total health promotion therapist might decide that the problem with the boy's rational field is the strategy, not the goal, and work on different strategies to achieve it. Alternatively, and this would be much more challenging, she might decide to work to change the prevailing environmental rational field, using the general foundations rational field template – hoping to achieve the most healthy school. Perhaps as pictured in **Figure 28**.

It no doubt seems quite unrealistic to suggest that the total health promoter should concentrate on the system rather than the individual (after all, it is infinitely easier to make the boy fit the system than the system fit the boy).

However, total health promotion must resist conventional assumptions. The basic premise of total health promotion is that we have got our classification systems wrong, or at least that which classification is the most health promoting is an open question. The total health promoter should not prejudge, but should display rational fields as they seem to be, and should work out what could happen given the application of the foundational rational field template.

The whole point of total health promotion is that nothing is fixed in stone and there is everything to play for – after all, health is at stake.

Of course, in reality – at least as things stand – the boy would be seen as the problem, and the total health promoter would probably have to go along with this. But this need not mean colluding with psychiatric classifications and drugs, since these are potentially damaging to the boy (especially the effects of drugs and the effect of being diagnosed with schizophrenia):

> All people suffer from one degree or another of mental helplessness in their routine lives. They need to collect their wits or regain their composure before proceeding with some difficult task. That is, they need to become rational and self-determined, and not helpless, despite their fears.[110]

Another way of putting this is that the total health promoter should help people create rational fields appropriate both to them and to the rational fields that surround them – and then work on making their chosen fields come to pass. Pretending that you are a famous boxer is not a good tactic because it cannot possibly fit within surrounding rational fields. But asking for protection from bullying and developing actual talents – even if they are not immediately valued by surrounding rational fields – is.[93]

This use of rational fields is a workable and realistic form of peace studies, and can be applied in all situations where two apparently incompatible rational fields co-exist with different degrees of power.

2. A situation where there is only one rational field permitted, A, and yet those who have to inhabit it have values and instincts which if given their head would not lead to the creation of rational field A but to other types of rational fields.

Assume that Rational Field A is created by a set of values p (ignore the other influencing factors, for simplicity):

A <------- Values p **A II** <-------Values q **A II** <------- Values r

II = barrier

In this case the person who must inhabit the field has values (q or r say) which would, ideally, be powerful enough to create an alternative rational field, but reality does not allow this. In reality only rational field **A** is possible. For example, parents and schools sometimes have different values with regard to religious norms (clothing, for instance) but only the school's rational field is possible. Or a parent wants to homeschool her child in preference to the mainstream schooling system, but for one reason or another has no alternative but to go along with the official option.

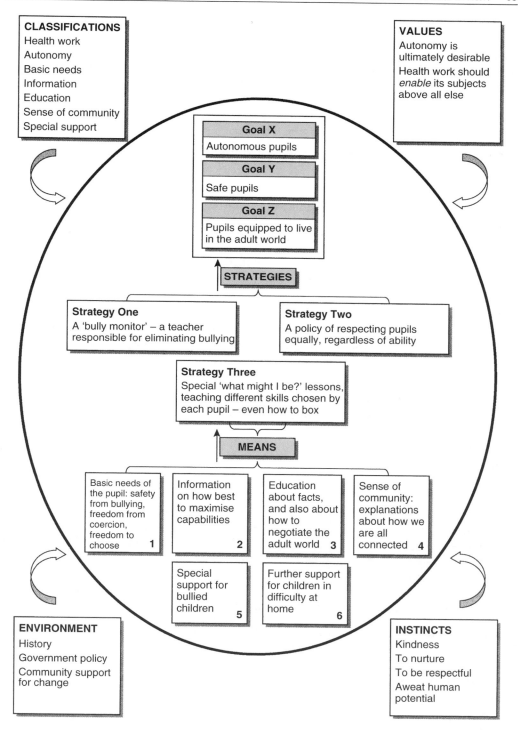

Figure 28 A possible strategy to achieve a healthier school using the General Foundations Rational Field Template

There are many well-known examples of this phenomenon that are dealt with by decision-makers who are openly sensitive to diverse values and goals. However there are also very many examples that are – by definition – hidden from most people's view. For example, here is a précised argument from a Maori Masters student, outlining Maori objections to the dominance of Western-based ethics committees:

DEVELOPING A MAORI PERSPECTIVE ON ETHICAL REVIEW IN [HEALTH] RESEARCH

Kaupapa Maori research has been at the forefront of an indigenous challenge to the research community and its traditional methodologies that have systematically objectivised and problematised Maori and Maori issues.[111]

(Note: In the words of a Maori educationalist responsible for codifying much of *kaupapa Maori* educational theory, 'kaupapa Maori research is research by Maori, for Maori and with Maori...'[112])

The proponents of Kaupapa Maori research recognised that some aspects of western research methodologies were inherently unethical when considered from a Maori point of view. They developed Kaupapa Maori research to address these concerns and have advocated approaches to research that are:

- more consistent with Maori beliefs and values
- focused on areas of Maori importance and concern
- going to result in some positive outcome for Maori
- controlled by Maori
- accountable to the community

and

- cognisant of Maori culture and preferences.

Despite the growing body of knowledge about Kaupapa Maori research and its application in a wide variety of fields, the ethical review process to which it is subjected is based on western philosophy. This has been a source of frustration for many Kaupapa Maori researchers who are asked to evaluate research projects designed to protect and enhance Maori values against principles based on western ones...This has become more evident in recent times with the strong emphasis on evidence-based practice (read research-based practice).

Ethical principles are set out as guides to the practice and behaviour of researchers to ensure that research is undertaken in ways to protect and enhance the interests of the participants...Ethical review in health research is guided by the Operational Standard for Ethics Committees.[113] It lists the guiding principles that govern the ethical review of proposals as:

- Respect for persons
- Informed consent
- Privacy and confidentiality

- Validity of research proposal
- Minimisation of harm
- Justice
- Cultural and social responsibility
- Compensation for research participants

...these principles...are substantially derived from the...western-oriented... ethical principles of autonomy, justice, beneficence and non-maleficence. The concepts of informed consent, privacy and confidentiality are bound by cultural notions...that first and foremost reside within the individual. However for cultures that promote collective autonomy over individual autonomy the concepts of individualised informed consent, privacy and confidentiality within the research process are a cultural nonsense...

...As processes, they are easier to assess than the sometimes vague notions of justice and beneficence which mean different things to different people. Subsequently these process oriented principles have seemingly become the primary focus of many ethics committees, while notions of justice and cultural responsibility, important motivators for any Maori researcher, are sidelined. While it is widely recognised that ethical principles can be contradictory in certain contexts, the hierarchical nature of their application (process principles over value principles) in ethical review has not been acknowledged. While I am sure this is unintended, it is a real experience and dilemma for many Maori researchers and Maori members of ethics committees. For example, the application form for gaining ethical approval from a Regional Health and Disability Ethics Committee has specific sections and questions for informed consent, confidentiality, research methods and compensation however there is no question regarding justice...[114]

The problem is obvious the moment this situation is depicted as a rational field plus causative factors. Even in the simplified form of **Figures 29** and **30**, were these images to be projected onto a screen at every ethics committee meeting, the committee members could not help but begin to think in very different ways.

To insist, as Western ethics committees insist to Maori, that it is perfectly fine for someone to inhabit an alien rational field is like commanding Wittgenstein's lion to become a retail worker in a shopping mall, or like telling a contented retail worker to become a lion in the jungle (it's possible but hardly desirable).

Once we can see these things properly revealed we can begin to decide what to do to improve matters – all of a sudden a host of new options is revealed. Certainly we can no longer sweep them under the carpet with any integrity.

3. A situation where there is supposedly a set of organisational values – rational field A – but where not all members of the organisation automatically create this rational field

For example, a teacher with an ethos of involving pupils in shared decision-making employed by a school with strict disciplinary standards will find herself in this situation.

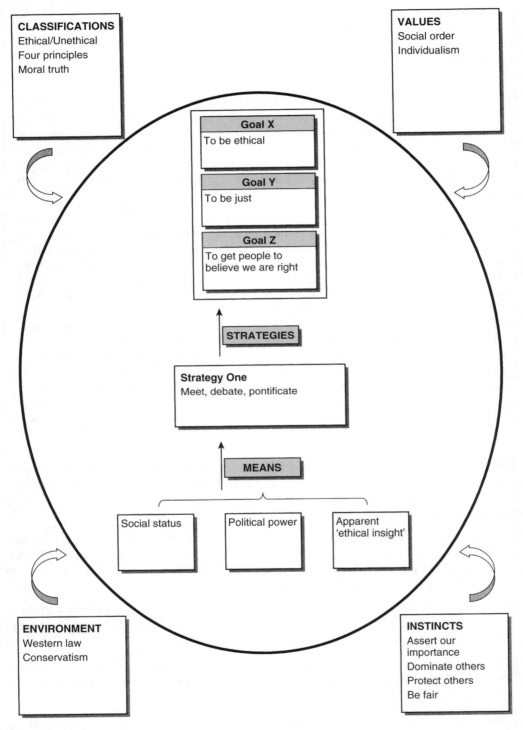

Figure 29   The Western Ethics Committee rational field

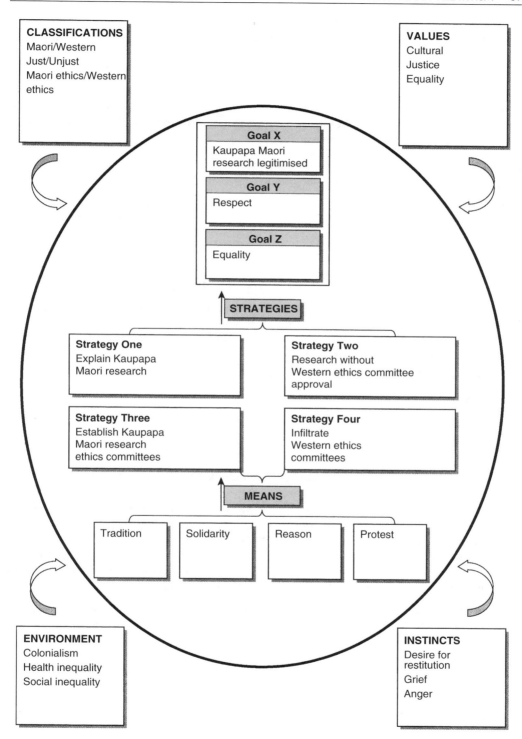

Figure 30   The Maori researchers' rational field

As will a humanitarian psychiatrist who chooses to ignore some diagnostic protocols in order to help his patients feel more valued. Seen from the perspective of the dominant rational field, it looks like the teacher and psychiatrist are subversives. However, once it is recognised that none of the rational fields can be regarded as ethically privileged, sensible debate about their differences can begin.

4. **A situation in which the values and instincts of the policy-makers would not create the Rational Field they have all agreed to: a rational elephant which no one really wants, designed by a committee**

In this situation, if it were possible for all members' rational fields to be laid out side by side – and alongside the official field – creative possibilities would abound.

In these circumstances, and 5 below, **VDM** software (or alternatives) could readily be used to help make difference in values and logic transparent (see **Chapter Four**).

5. **Micro-situations where a single choice (agree/disagree) has to be made but there are many different values and forms of reasoning in play.**

As we shall see (in **Chapter 4**), by using **VDM** software it is possible:

- To reveal a range of values, instincts and classifications
- To consider the different logical approaches which each generates
- To recognise that if one verdict has to be sustained then at least all the dissenting notions should remain visible, in a 'values rich' environment

6. **A situation where the rational field is not correctly expressed**

For example:

- By mistake
- By oversimplification
- By subterfuge

Revealing the actual values and instincts would show that the apparent rational field is mistaken. For example, say that the prevailing policy in a mental illness institution is 'seclusion'. By using the rational field template with participation from all interested parties, it is possible to show how many people's values sets create the seclusion policy rational field, and how many do not. One way to do this would be to see how people who don't espouse the seclusion rational field 'build' alternative fields. Another method would be to show that the values even of those who say they espouse the seclusion field don't lead to it, or also lead to alternative fields/policies.

7. **A situation where the relationship between the inner parts and outer elements of existing fields are investigated in order to try to detect the real reasons for outcomes and trends**

For example, it is well known that more black people are involuntarily detained than white:

> African-Caribbean people are six times more likely than whites to be diagnosed as schizophrenic, but research shows this is nothing to do with biology. A study by the Institute of Psychiatry has found that poor social conditions are causing black people to develop the symptoms of mental illness.
>
> The high rates of black people inside Britain's psychiatric system has concerned both the medical profession, and the black community for many years.

And the government's mental health czar admitted the mental health system is institutionally racist.

Questioned on BBC Two's *Newsnight*, National Director of Mental Health, Professor Louis Appleby, said: If by that you mean that the system operates to the disadvantage of some racial groups, I have no doubt about that. . . .

Researchers from the Institute of Psychiatry investigated whether black people were somehow genetically more prone to schizophrenia.

The answer was no – they found rates among black people in the Caribbean were identical to the white population to the UK.[115]

and

Research has shown that the mental health needs of the African-Caribbean community would be better met if there existed a more culturally appropriate service available, staffed by culturally competent health professionals. This would require educational knowledge with a multi-cultural and multi-ethnic perspective from the initial training stage for health care professionals. In addition, any equal opportunity policies implemented to engender this approach should be regularly evaluated to ensure that the needs of the minority ethnic populations are being effectively met.[116]

The Spock-bubble part of this situation is simple enough – a problem arises, the normal psychiatric processes kick in, it is defined as a personal problem of mental illness, a person is treated. Now, taking a sample of black and white patients it becomes possible to compare and contrast outer decision sources for treating black and white patients – are the professionals' values and instincts different for black and white people, and does this give us a more realistic picture than looking only at the inner rational field?

My educated guess is that it might.

OBJECTIONS TO THE RATIONAL FIELD APPROACH

Inevitably, there are objections to the rational field approach. For example:

Question: Doesn't the rational field view lead to the fragmentation of the self? If each individual is composed of billions of natural and manufactured rational fields, what is left of the individual *per se*? If lungs, and tissues and cells and atoms and electrical impulses are each rational fields then doesn't the idea of a human person simply disintegrate?

Answer: No, of course not. I'm writing this and you are reading it. I haven't disintegrated (yet) and nor have you. This is because our rational fields are held together in vastly complex and mutually supporting hierarchies.[105] Rational fields are rarely if ever independent and free-floating. Rather they exist in context – and the rational fields which make up we human beings exist in the context of society, intent, identity, belief in the self, history and so on. Human rational fields are organised through automatic physical function (the heart pumping blood, the blood distributing oxygen and so on) and also through intentional organisation – I will my body to play a game of squash because I temporarily create a rational field with the goals leisure, exercise, fun, comradeship and (in moments of wild optimism) victory. As I will this, millions of other rational fields are briefly created and then disappear (increased endorphin levels and distribution, a psychological ploy as I take an unneeded drink break just as my opponent is about to serve for the game ☺, that sweeping backhand winner, and so on).

Question: Doesn't the rational field approach simply take us right back to relativism?

Answer: No, because seeing the world as made up of billions of rational fields shows us how much we share. Millions of our rational fields are held entirely in common (in particular those which emanate from our urge to classify the world, our instincts, our preferences and our physical and social environments – everyone has rules, rituals, celebrations, feeding times, happy times, grieving times), millions are sometimes shared and sometimes not (belief in some form of the supernatural for example) and millions are in conflict (the aspirations of three people to gain a single job, the desire of a mother both to protect her child and to encourage her independence, my wish to be fit and my wish to use alcohol to relax, the belief that it is right to go to war for a cause and the belief that only pacifism can be justified).

By recognising this magnificent multiplicity of rational fields we can see how we are part of everything, we can see how much we share with other creatures, we can change ourselves, we can try to change others, we can try to understand ourselves, we can try to understand others, we can try to understand the world outside ourselves – and we can explicitly try to change it in ways we believe are for the better.

It is even possible to ease into other people's rational fields, and to do so knowingly. You can try out what they do and can try to see things as they do – of course you cannot be them but you can try to be like them, at least experimentally (this is a very familiar concept to novelists and playwrights). The rational field approach is about stepping back and thinking about reason and purpose rather than being driven by it, it is about stepping back and feeling that you have feelings, and about recognising their force on your Spock-reason. The rational field approach is not about seeing other people, cultures and the external as alien and unreachable. Rather it is about tolerance – more than anything else it is about tolerance.

Question: Isn't the idea of rational fields merely a description of something everyone knows already?

Answer: I hope so.

HOW TO UNDERSTAND WITTGENSTEIN'S LION

To help sum up this possibly rather difficult chapter, recall the three case studies at its head, and the mammography example. Each case contains miscomprehension between people who see the same evidence in different ways. In each case, there is apparently no connection – other than the evidence – between the different parties' understandings. The senior committee members even try to explain their behaviours to the student representative. He hears their words, but though everyone is speaking English, he cannot make sense of what they say. It seems to him that they are playing an absurd game and have their priorities bizarrely wrong.

This is probably what Wittgenstein meant when he wrote:

> If a lion could talk, we could not understand him[69]

Just before this oft-quoted pronouncement, Wittgenstein explained:

> We also say of some people that they are transparent to us. It is, however, important as regards this observation that one human being can be a complete enigma to another. We

learn this when we come into a strange country with entirely strange traditions; and, what is more, even given a mastery of the country's language. We do not *understand* the people. (And not because of not knowing what they are saying to themselves.) We cannot find our feet with them . . .

If a lion could talk, we could not understand him.[69]

The inability to *find our feet* with other people is a more accessible way of accounting for our frequent failure to see the point of other people's traditions, words and behaviours. Either we just don't get them at all, or we interpret other people's expressions in our own terms, distorting their meanings. The student representative at the committee meeting could not find his feet with his new colleagues and they could not find their feet with him.

I think Wittgenstein was implying that it is simply foreignness that does this. He believed that in order to understand other people you have to be saturated in the way they live – immersed in their 'form of life', as he put it. You have to LIVE these other people's meanings rather than merely read them in a book, or learn about them from a tour guide while on holiday.

The same applies to the tourist on the bridge, the artist creating the shell picture, and the different committees trying to decide whether or not to recommend mammography for women in their forties. The tourist cannot understand the citizens of Safe Harbour because he doesn't live in the place and in the ways they do. If he spoke to them of his idea for a vast aquatic transport system they would hear his words but they would not take him seriously. He would be like a lion to them.

The artist can see her picture of Glory as plainly as she can see her hand in front of her face, but her friend sees nothing because she has not given him even a clue about how to step into her way of seeing the world. They could talk about the shells, and yet even when she had shown him the pattern he still may not see the point of it as she does, simply because he had not had the experiences and thoughts that led her to craft it that way.

My most repeated personal experience of dealing with lions has been my academic encounters with members of the psychiatry profession (which is one reason why so many of my examples are taken from psychiatry). They talk to me, but I cannot understand them, even though I've read the books they read, worked with them as colleagues and have been awarded university degrees from the same system that awarded them their degrees. To me, psychiatry is a cruel and conceptually baseless pseudo-profession – a house of cards lacking even one plausible definition of its key terms, and possessing not a shred of decent theory about its purpose. Psychiatry exists, I assume, as a way of removing potentially detrimental people from society, and a means of maintaining the social status quo. And yet I am also aware that tens of thousands of people just as sensitive and intelligent as I are psychiatrists, and that the system has withstood intense scrutiny and criticism over the last forty years. So, I assume, I am just unable to see something that is completely clear to the psychiatrists.

If we want to understand ourselves better the challenge for all of us is to become accomplished in thinking of the world as made up of rational fields, in order to explore ways of understanding our lions. Although I cannot comprehend how Robert the psychiatrist can poison other people's children with Ritalin, I can instantly understand his love for his own children, and we can have the deepest talks about the soccer team we both support.

Once we recognise that all 'other lions' have innumerable rational fields then maybe we can find ways to expose their geneses in ways every lion can understand. Indeed, it may ultimately be possible using simple language, graphic representations and choices, to expose all lions' rational fields for open scrutiny: possibly through the **VDM** software explained in the next chapter.

CHAPTER FOUR

How to Turn Values into Evidence

Psychologists long have known that people make decisions based on emotion and then justify the decision with other reasons born of logic. However, in the new millennium, there will be less need to validate emotion. Intuition is no longer scorned and scoffed at – rather, it is valued.[117]

SUMMARY

- If lions are to talk to each other we need a method to bring them together meaningfully – values-based decision-making (**VDM**) is a highly promising way forward
- Practical **VDM** must avoid the dead-end approach
- **VDM** is best understood as a way to achieve decision transparency
- The groundbreaking VIDe project to build **VDM** software is described
- A range of potential objections to **VDM** are tackled

———————————— ◆ ————————————

Because all decision making involves values, all decision-making is values-based decision-making. However, there are two contrasting inspirations for **VDM** – one with amazing potential, the other a dead-end.

ASSUMING THAT THE RIGHT VALUES ARE OBVIOUS: THE DEAD-END APPROACH TO VDM

The belief in right and wrong is fundamental to the human sense of purpose and hope. When people first hear the phrase 'values-based decision-making', they mostly imagine an approach based on 'right values' – like 'family values', 'caring values' or 'business values'. For example:

> Workplace values are the standards we set for our interactions with our clients and with each other. They include such things as serving the public interest, excellence, team-work, integrity and compassion. Ethics is the way we put our values to work in actual decision-making – that is, in doing the right thing.[118]

> A values-based approach to business ethics helps sort out the positive values that need to be encouraged from those that need to be rooted out. The result will be a culture that expresses positive values and creates a climate that supports ethical and legal decision-making.[119]

Unfortunately perhaps, it is highly naïve to believe in a simple right/wrong or positive/negative values dichotomy. One person's positive values may be another person's negative values, and such notions as 'integrity', the 'public interest' and 'excellence' are very obviously open to wide interpretation.

'Health values' are sometimes referred to as obviously right values.[120] For example:

> If we ask ourselves why we believe in having healthcare, we can answer perhaps that we need it to prevent and relieve human suffering, and to prevent untimely death. Then we can ask why we want these preventions, and answer that suffering is intrinsically bad, because it represents negative, destructive experience, and that untimely death is wasteful and a denial of potential. If we question why these things matter, we are forced to fall back on very general arguments about the intrinsic value of individual human life in quantity and quality, about human security and flourishing, about the values of living in stable and supportive communities. When we ask why these things are important, we realise that we have come to an end of reason. We can only reply that life can be no other way, that individuals and societies cannot flourish without the sense of security that comes from an acceptance that individual human life has significance, both for our own lives and the unique, individual lives of others. These are the sorts of values that ultimately underpin the health endeavour. They justify, for example, the principles of principle-based ethics in medicine, the principles of respect for the autonomy of others, of beneficence, non-maleficence and justice. Principles do not simply emerge from nowhere. They are based on values and beliefs....[121]

It is true that 'principles do not simply emerge from nowhere'. However, closer examination of Little's statement is revealing. In short, he says:

1. Suffering is bad
2. Human security and flourishing, and living in stable and supportive communities are good
3. We cannot use reason to say why these things (at **2**) are important
4. These things (at **2**) are important because life can be no other way
5. The values (at **1** and **2**) ultimately underpin the health endeavour
6. The values (at **1** and **2**) justify the principles of medical ethics
7. Principles are based on values

Let's take these statements in turn:

1 is arguable. If it means ALL suffering is bad then on reflection hardly anyone would agree with it – we need to experience SOME suffering to learn, to grow and to feel sympathy for other peoples' suffering. The best we can say is that for some people, in some circumstances, suffering is not wanted (though there are religions – Buddhism for example – that urge us to welcome and embrace suffering of all kinds).

There is always room for debate where values are concerned. However, because we are so used to our own preferences we tend to assume other people hold them too, or if they don't that they should hold them if they want to be right-thinking.

2 is vague and therefore not obvious – vague statements look obvious because they are vague (their vagueness conceals a range of possible meanings and we cannot know which of these meanings the writer intends).

If we assume specific meanings for the expressions at **2** then the statement is clearly arguable. For example:

... individuals and societies cannot flourish without the sense of security that comes from an acceptance that individual human life has significance ...[121]

But what sort of security should we value? The sort of security that means putting armed police officers on commercial flights? The sort of security that builds walls between nations (as in Israel in 2004) and barbed wire on walls around houses (as in South Africa for decades). Or some other sort of security – perhaps the security of knowing that one can leave one's house unlocked and not lose any possessions (in which case hardly anyone these days has such security)?

What sort of flourishing is good? Rebellious exultation? Conformity to the values and expectations of elders? Obedience at school even if it means taking Ritalin for years?

3 Is false. Not only can we use reason to say why the things at **2** are important, we must do so in a world where there is a plurality of values and where all value-statements are open to a range of interpretations. Values-based decision-making is not just about preferences – it is about giving and sustaining reasons for those preferences.

4 Is false. The statement that 'life can be no other way' is an attempt to convince without argument, and it is of course a false statement. Life can be other ways – many other ways – and frequently is.

5 Is arguable. Firstly, which specific meanings/values underpin the 'health endeavour'? Secondly, what is the health endeavour? The nature of the 'health endeavour' is not obvious – there are many alternative understandings of health, some of which are in conflict. 'Health' is an evaluative term, not a scientific one.[81]

6 Is false. Values cannot justify principles without circularity because principles are themselves values. The reason some bioethicists like to use the principle 'respect autonomy' is simply because respecting other people's choices is one of their preferences.

7 Is true. However, the perpetually open question is whether the values – and therefore the principles – are worth anything.

Little goes on to discuss his understanding of 'values-based medicine'. He says:

> At the deepest level, our values, both personal and societal, justify and sustain the medical endeavour. If we, in Western societies, did not place so high a value on individual human life in quantity and quality, we would rebel against the huge expenditures we commit to health services. Would it therefore be better to use 'values-based' medicine as our therapeutic term rather than the somewhat unsatisfactory 'humanistic' medicine? There are certainly arguments in favour of values-based medicine.
>
> First and foremost, the term invites us to remember the ultimate, sustaining values-base for healthcare services. We *do* value individual human life. It is this value that justifies personal medicine, and public health services. The health of communities reflects the health of their individual members ...
>
> Third, and most importantly, values-based medicine seeks to go beyond any reductionist model, because it asks that we consult our values when we face dilemmas and problems of service delivery. It does not seek to reduce medicine to one of its components. Our values underpin all those component parts, and each component becomes important as a means of expressing those values.[121]

Little's dificulties of reasoning occur because he believes these underpinning values are obvious. When he says:

> If we, in Western societies, did not place so high a value on individual human life in quantity and quality, we would rebel against the huge expenditures we commit to health services ...

he merely assumes that this is true. But it is unclear how many people realise how much taxpayers' money is spent on medical care (do you know?). Nor is it clear how many people are bothered about medical expenditure, or would be bothered were they to know about it. Certainly the general public is rarely directly asked for an opinion on this question. To my knowledge, no government has ever asked us if we would prefer more money spent on efforts to guarantee full and fulfilling employment for all citizens and less on high-tech hospitals. We do not know very well what people's values are about this complex matter; we surely cannot conclude that just because a social institution exists, it is universally valued, or indeed valued in the same way by everyone.

Little says, 'We *do* value individual human life.' And of course we do. How could we not? However, there are real questions about how much we value human life (what is a human life worth?);[122] how we value different human lives; and how we balance individual human lives against broader social priorities – governments could reduce the influence of fast-food giants on children's eating habits through legislation in advertising and nutritional quality, but they don't; governments could reduce road accidents by enforcing 70 kph maximum speeds in cars, but they don't.

Little also says, 'It is this value that justifies personal medicine, and public health services.' But only careful reasoning can justify decisions (like decisions about how to invest in medical services) that favour some people ahead of others – vague values held by some people but not all people are neither foolproof nor satisfactory justifications on any sensible understanding of 'justify'.

DECISION SUPPORT

If 'decision-support' is the provision of evidence, experience and knowledge to assist decision-making, then it is possible to think of **VDM** as decision support. For example, **VDM** can:

- Strengthen people's confidence by revealing shared values (as people see that others think as they do)
- Support people to find ways to apply their values in a practical and structured way to solve problems
- Support people to see the merits of other people's values (and rational fields)

However, while there are overlaps between decision-support systems and decision-transparency systems (making decision processes transparent can obviously bring about better practical decision-making), **VDM's** primary motivation is to clarify values, their relationship to evidence, and the influence of both on decision-making.

DECISION TRANSPARENCY

There are already many ways – both technical and commonplace – to render people's values transparent.

Technical approaches to decision transparency include:

- Opinion polls
- Market surveys
- Economic surveys, such as willingness-to-pay

- Deliberative mapping
- Psychological tests
- Psychotherapy
- Polygraphs (lie detectors)
- Political elections[123-130]

Each of these is interested in what people believe and feel, and how their beliefs and feelings affect their behaviour.

Commonplace approaches to decision transparency include:

- Observing what people do
- Observing how people spend their money
- Getting people drunk (*in vino veritas*)
- Taking people to court and asking them to tell the truth on oath
- Employing a private investigator to find out what people say and do when they think no one is watching them
- Simply asking people to tell you what they think

EXPLICITLY VALUES-BASED DECISION-TRANSPARENCY SYSTEMS

The ultimate purpose of each of the above decision-transparency systems, technical and commonplace, is to make preferences clear. However, there are currently only a handful of non-dead-end projects EXPLICITLY devoted to values-based decision-making, and almost all of these have distinct limitations:

> Given a particular decision context and a decision maker with a set of personal values, it may be very difficult to see all sides of the issue. Yet, being able to view the decision environment from multiple perspectives would enhance the decision maker's ability to make better-informed choices.

> ... the Value-Based Decision-Making (**VBDM**) model (suggests) that multiple perspectives may be achieved by considering a foundation of individual values... This model provides a framework that decision-makers and researchers can use to better understand and facilitate the use of multiple perspectives in decision-making and organizational memory enhancement.[131]

The authors of the above extract clearly appreciate the importance of viewing 'the decision environment from multiple perspectives', yet remain a fair way off coming up with a practical way to do this.

The creators of an interesting engineering and building example argue:

> Decisions made by multiple collaborating parties often involve *conflicts* among preferences, i.e., different parties prefer different options. Person A may prefer glazing option 1 because of its aesthetic appeal while person B may prefer glazing option 2 because of its superior energy performance. The final decision is made by the most powerful player(s) in the decision-making process who is generally influenced by the debate. (p. 4)[132]

They describe a model for the 'integration of multiple processes' but admit that 'significant work' is needed to turn this into a working tool. Similarly, the UA Center for Integral Leadership recognises that:

> Today's economic climate poses many leadership challenges including driving change. Change raises ethical issues because it is based on organizational values. Since these common values determine the choice of goals to be managed and measured, leaders must determine these values in order to be successful. ActionPoint and the UACIL

provide an anonymous environment in which values are shared without fear of reprisal and management can actually measure performance gains. Through this joint process of integrating values, leaders build trust within their team and can demonstrate the results.[133]

Again, however, there is little practical clarity about how to assess and balance values in a practically useful way.

THE FULFORD APPROACH

Psychiatrist and philosopher Bill Fulford has a long-standing interest in the philosophical and practical analysis of health care. Consequently, he recognises the importance of clarifying and building upon the values inevitably in play in health care situations. In his words:

> Values-Based Practice (**VBP**) is the theory and practice of effective healthcare decision-making for situations in which legitimately different (and hence potentially conflicting) value perspectives are in play.

> As a theory, **VBP** is the values-counterpart of Evidence-Based Practice, or **EBP**. **VBP** and **EBP** are both responses to the growing complexity of decision-making in healthcare: **EBP** is a response to the growing complexity of the relevant facts; **VBP** is a response to the growing complexity of the relevant values.[134]

Fulford outlines ten principles of values-based practice:

The Theory

1st Principle of **VBP**
- All decisions stand on two feet, on values as well as on facts, including decisions about diagnosis

2nd Principle of **VBP**
- We tend to notice values only when they are diverse or conflicting and hence are likely to be problematic

3rd Principle of **VBP**
- Scientific progress, in opening up choices, is increasingly bringing the full diversity of human values into play in all areas of healthcare

4th Principle of **VBP**
- **VBP's** 'first call' for information is the perspective of the patient or patient group concerned in a given decision

5th Principle of **VBP**
- In **VBP**, conflicts of values are resolved primarily, not by reference to a rule prescribing a 'right' outcome, but by processes designed to support a balance of legitimately different perspectives

The Practice

6th Principle of **VBP**
- Careful attention to language use in a given context is one of a range of powerful methods for raising awareness of values

7th Principle of **VBP**
- A rich resource of both empirical and philosophical methods is available for improving our knowledge of other people's values

8th Principle of **VBP**
- Ethical reasoning is employed in **VBP** primarily to explore differences of values, not, as in quasi-legal bioethics, to determine 'what is right'

9th Principle of **VBP**
- In **VBP**, communication skills have a substantive rather than (as in quasi-legal ethics) a merely executive role in clinical decision-making

10th Principle of **VBP**
- **VBP**, although involving a partnership with ethicists and lawyers (equivalent to the partnership with scientists and statisticians in **EBP**), puts decision-making back where it belongs, with users and providers at the clinical coal-face[135]

Though they can currently be advanced only through labour-intensive workshops, Fulford's principles are a thoughtful and accessible backcloth to the development of time-efficient values-based decision-making systems for practice.

THE VIDE SOFTWARE PROJECT (©VIDE LTD)

The VIDe project has come about through philosophy and the desire to use it to change the world.

The point of philosophy is to improve our lives by bringing about increased clarity of understanding. There is no reason why philosophical activity should be confined to learned journals and university seminar rooms. Consequently, my colleagues and I have developed an interactive software decision-transparency system designed to bring values-based decision-making fully into the practical realm.

The system is founded in part upon the theoretical assumptions explained in the first three chapters of this book, and on two previously published decision-making tools (the Rings of Uncertainty and the Ethical Grid[77]). It could not have been invented without this philosophical background.

This system does not tell you which values are best or right or true or objective, nor does it instruct users to apply particular values to solve particular problems. Rather the VIDe version of **VDM** exposes all value-judgements (in the context of as much evidence as possible) for scrutiny by all who are making them and all who have an interest in them.

Other practically minded philosophers are equally enthusiastic about this goal:

> ... decisions are most effective when they incorporate clearly identified values.
>
> Values, or those qualities we deem useful, develop from our backgrounds and experience, from family and peers, culture, profession and religion.
>
> Virtually all our choices and decisions are values-based. When we make a difficult choice, we do so because certain values matter more than others.
>
> It may be the "bottom line in business," our need for job security, legal constraints, a sense of obligation to tell the truth, honoring a commitment to keep promises, loyalty to a friend or co-worker, a deep respect for the importance of our family ties or compassion for others.
>
> It isn't a matter of whether values such as these come into play. They do.
>
> How able are we, then, to clearly name all our own values and to elicit and clarify those of others that are embedded in important decisions? How skilled are we in working with a number of applicable values, in sorting and weighing these values, so that we use those we understand to be most important to make difficult choices and drive our decisions? ...
>
> The skills we need desperately involve understanding and discerning how to choose when a decision will honor some values that matter, while failing to honor, even violating other values that also matter.

"Values talk" makes many people nervous, however.

In business settings it can signal an endless discussion that goes nowhere. In social and political arenas it may be used to set some above others to judge them – usually negatively. In less formal, more personal conversations, we may be reluctant to "impose our values on others." The goal of productive dialogue with those whose values seem so different, perhaps opposite, from our own seems like an impossible dream.

Yet the desire somehow to find "higher ground" and civility as we tackle tough issues in our public, business and personal lives seems only to grow. As does the recognition that we need to find ways to honor important values and principles while respecting differences, building bridges that bring people together instead of driving wedges among us …

Here are some of the highlights of what we consider to be an effective, values-based decision making process, from the perspective of those whose place it is to decide:

- FRAMING: The decision maker is aware of her or his point of view – frame – on this issue. What kind of an issue do you think it is? For example, do you think of it as "business" decision, a "policy" decision, an "engineering" decision, a "strategic" decision, a "human resources" decision, a "legal" decision? These labels may limit what values are considered relevant or highlight certain values as key. They may also blind us to impacts on others. What assumptions are you making about the issue?

- NAMING: What values do you bring to this issue? What do you think is important to consider? Are you willing and able to speak up about the organizational, professional, or personal values that matter to you in this context?

- CLARIFYING: What values do others bring to the issue? Have you listened well to what they believe matters? Have you, too, been heard and understood? Are you satisfied that all the applicable values have been identified and explained clearly?

- WEIGHING: Among these identified values, which ones rise to the top in importance in this situation? Have you identified all the options that should be considered? Is there an option that honors all or most of the top values?

- DECIDING: What decision clearly follows from these identified top values?

- REPORTING: Are you prepared to communicate the decision based on the values that drove it? Who deserves to hear about the choice you made? Are you willing and able to acknowledge and be accountable for those values that also mattered but could not be honored in the decision? Can you describe the reasons for weighing some values as more important than others in this situation?

Good decision makers are clear, deliberate, and reflective. They can explain, and if necessary, justify their decisions. They have thought through the basis for the decision and its consequences. They are role models for us, because they know what they believe is important and their decisions are authentically based on these values.[136]

The VIDe system for **VDM** has been constructed in this spirit.

A BRIEF INTRODUCTION TO THE VIDE SYSTEM (WWW.VIDE.CO.NZ)

The VIDe system (for healthcare providers) divides participating professionals into user groups (for example, Learning Disabilities, Obstetrics, Psychiatric Nursing, and so on). On request from any user the case administrator for a particular group posts a case (which may be linked into electronic patient record systems) for consideration by the rest of the team. For example, see **Figure 31**.

The user can access the case notes (**Figure 32**).

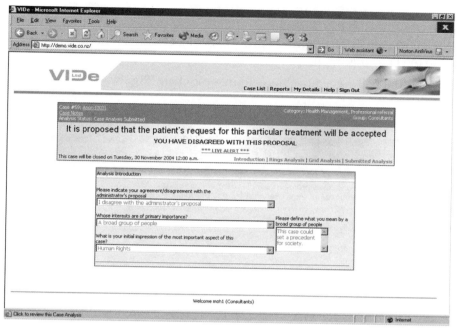

Figure 31

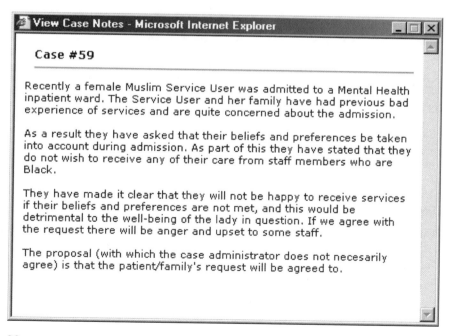

Figure 32

He or she can then agree or disagree with the proposal, state whose interests are of primary importance, and give an initial impression of the most important aspect of the case (this has already been done in **Figure 31** above). Once she's done this, the user can proceed to the Perception Rings.

At this screen she will see a movable, coloured pie chart (**Figure 33**).

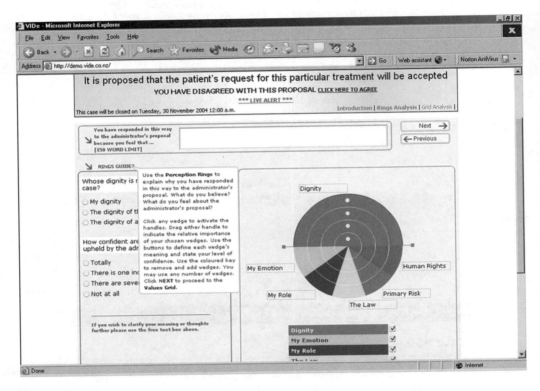

Figure 33

This screen enables the user to give a gut reaction (for want of a better term) to the administrator's proposal. Using it, she can say how she feels as a human being about what is being suggested. Once she has expressed herself using the pie chart she will end up with something resembling **Figure 34.**

The user may then proceed to the Values Grid where she can put forward an argument about what she thinks should be done. By clicking on various tiles and using free text she can engage in ethical analysis and make suggestions about how to proceed. She will come up with an image something like **Figure 35**.

Once she's happy that this is the best argument she can present, the user can proceed to the final screen, where she will be reminded of any inconsistencies in her thinking and where she can post any final thoughts and explanations she may have (**Figure 36**).

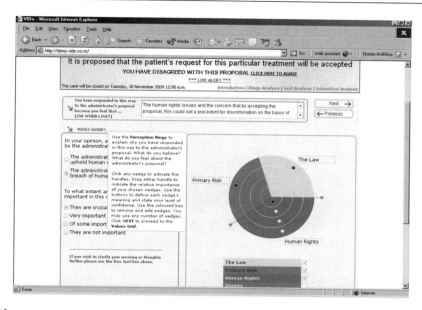

Figure 34

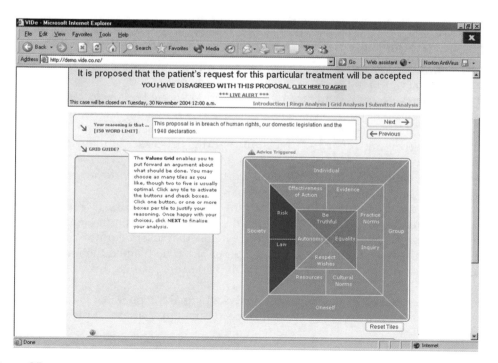

Figure 35

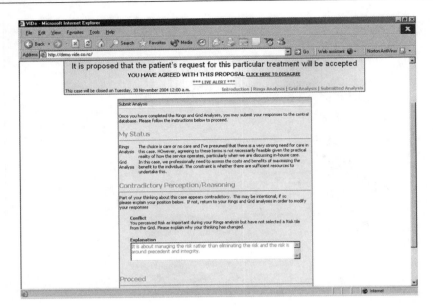

Figure 36
(Note: **Figures 31–36** show different users' analyses)

Her information is now secure within the VIDe database. It can be added to and compared with data from other users in order to produce multiple patterns of use, and insights into values trends. For example see **Figures 37** to **41**.

These reports instantly reveal important trends, consensus and conflict.

In sum, the VIDe system:

- Systematically reveals and clarifies the human values, preferences and biases that are part of all decision-making
- Unites values-based and evidence-based decision-making
- Creates an extensive audit trail of values-based decision-making previously unavailable to clinicians, management, health insurers and patients
- Provides a growing record of decision-making processes, linked to electronic clinical data
- Offers unique reporting functions designed to enhance policy development, quality assurance, ethical audit, peer review and risk-management
- Provides live alerts, crucial for highlighting unspoken conflict/lack of consensus, and for preventing misunderstandings exploding into conflict and damage.
- Provides compulsory action alerts which mean that users cannot continue their analyses until they have either changed their choice or explained their actions. These are crucial for ensuring that controversial decisions are justified by legal or research references
- Supports personal education in values analysis by making personal values explicit to each user, and by revealing personal decision-making patterns, consistencies and inconsistencies

For further information about VIDe systems contact: info@vide.co.nz. To join a growing international network of values-based decision-making, visit values-exchange.com.

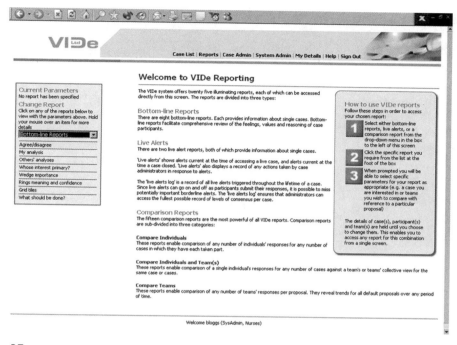

Figure 37

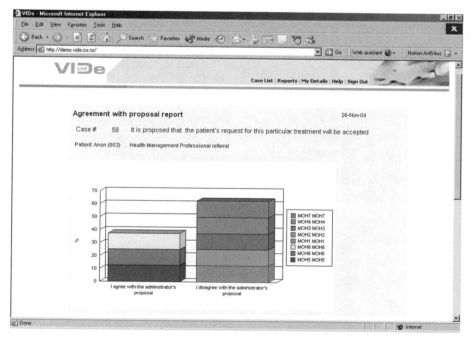

Figure 38

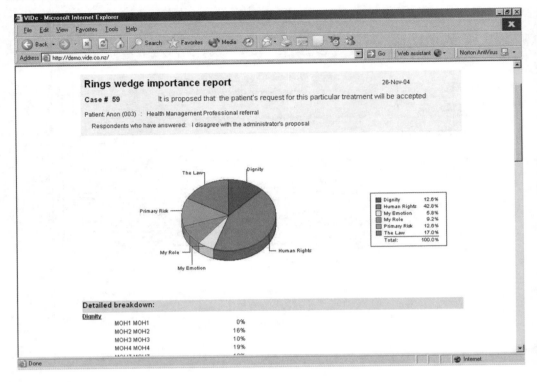

Figure 39

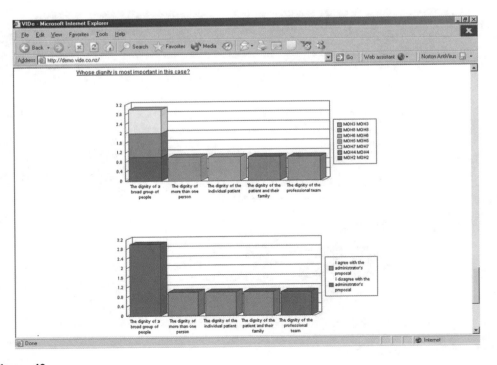

Figure 40

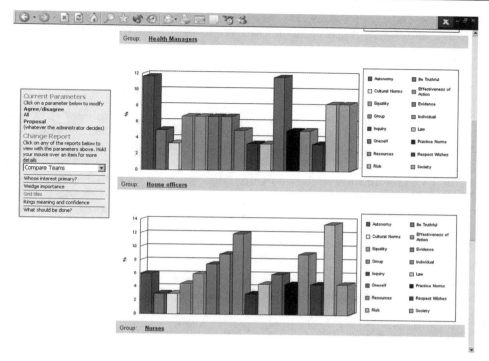

Figure 41

POTENTIAL OBJECTIONS TO VALUES-BASED DECISION-MAKING SOFTWARE

VDM IS NOT PHILOSOPHICALLY PERFECT

There is no doubt that a competent philosopher could drive a coach and horses through every aspect of the VIDe project (as a qualified philosopher myself, I can say this with some confidence). However, this certainly does not mean that **VDM** is not a workable idea.

In order to build a practical way to elicit people's feelings and arguments about life problems, compromises are necessary. Analytic philosophy requires that every statement about anything must be defined, reasoned and justified. Philosophy seeks to refine meanings and distinctions as far as they can go. For example, to satisfy a strict philosopher the nature of 'dignity' or 'rights' or 'risk' (part of the Perception Rings) must be identified well beyond the extent of the current software.[137] The distinction between 'preferences' and 'reasoning' – which is taken for granted by the software – could undoubtedly be disputed. And the many reports the system generates could each be dissected and challenged. To a purist philosopher, the meaning of say:

> I feel positive emotions toward the individual patient

Or:

> Damage to my integrity or to the organisation's integrity

will look hopelessly vague. And I mean hopelessly. I am entirely aware that the nature of 'positive emotion' is highly disputable. At the very least we need a list of those things that are deemed to count as positive – and indeed, of those things that are to count as emotional states at all. Is 'warmth' a positive emotion? If so, does the TYPE of warmth count? If a health professional feels sexual desire toward the recipient of his care, and is motivated by this, is this a positive or negative emotion?

And what does 'integrity' mean? Is my view of my integrity a valid one? How, in the absence of any general notion of 'integrity', can I even tell (there is nothing about this within the tools)? Integrity might mean: wholeness, being true to oneself, being true to given standards, being respectful of other people's beliefs. And – from a philosophical point of view – each of these ideas, sooner or later, is bound to conflict with each of the others. If I'm true to myself then I may go against a socially accepted standard, or I may decide that being true to myself means explicitly not respecting some other person's beliefs, for one reason or another. Perhaps my understanding of integrity includes the idea of tolerance and I find that some other people have views that are intolerant – so I may then decide not to be tolerant of their intolerance.

It is really very easy to be a philosopher critic. And yet it is unquestionably important that we can obtain some sort of idea about the evaluative components of decision-making.

What are we to do? Do we abandon a system that may give us useful insights into values trends, and may even bring about a more reflective culture (and partly BECAUSE many of its meanings are open to interpretation) just because some of its meanings are vague and might produce an out-of-focus picture of what is going on? Or do we bite the bullet and build systems which plainly have both practical and philosophical limitations, trying to get from them those things we can reasonably hope to get from them? Do we make a start and hope to improve as we go on, or do we abandon the whole project as philosophically flawed?

There is no question that it IS philosophically flawed – the issue is, is it so philosophically flawed that it is of no use at all?

Clearly the existing system can provide useful (if sometimes blurry) information about the ways people think about what they do. In addition it can help us recognise:

- The limits of our daily conversations
- The limits of codes of practice
- The current limits of health professional education
- The need for SOME system to render decision-making more transparent – even if it is not this one
- The constant and inescapable presence of values

POSSIBLE GENERAL LIMITATIONS OF ATTEMPTS TO ACHIEVE VALUES TRANSPARENCY

The general problems confronting **VDM** seem to be as follows.

Values change in different contexts

It is not possible to say with certainty that *Value X* is one of Billy's values because he may not hold this value in every circumstance. For example, Billy might mostly value 'being kind to strangers' and would usually stop to help someone fallen by the roadside.

But not always. Sometimes – maybe when he is feeling angry or depressed or more self-centred than usual – Billy might just walk on by.[138] Even if Billy's reasons are taken into account (i.e. he might have good reasons not to be a Good Samaritan in some circumstances) it remains true that people's hierarchies of values are not always consistent, and are continually subject to reordering by external factors.

But if this is the reality then it isn't a problem for **VDM**. It merely means that we should be very careful to take context into account, and be wary of making abstract or general statements about people's values.

This will be equally so if it turns out that people's values change even in the same contexts (i.e. if they decide one way one day and another way the next in the same circumstances). If a person's values change like this, the question is why? Perhaps the person is growing with experience, is learning, is thoughtful and open-minded. Maybe more consistent types – people whose values remain constant – are TOO inflexible.

The meanings of values words are hard to pin down and communicate accurately

The meanings of values words are open to wide interpretation. For example, what one person means by 'the common good' might not be what her colleague means by it – one might mean 'increased profit', the other might mean 'better health'. And these additional notions require exploration and definition in turn – what sort of profit? What sort of health?

People may not give true answers

There are at least five possible problems in this regard:

1. Making mistakes using the system

Users of the VIDe system might:

- Accidentally select unintended categories (they might, for example, fail to size wedges to reflect correctly what they mean)
- Interpret any of the system's questions to mean something other than the system designer envisaged
- Interpret proposals to mean something other than the proposer intends

To some extent these effects are inevitable, and are seen in actual uses of the software. However, they are reduced by:

- Training
- Practice
- Peer review
- Continuing improvements to the clarity of the proposals and questions with experience

2. Deliberate dishonesty

There are certain pressures on honesty with values-based decision-transparency systems. Primarily these are:

- Embarrassment about expressing one's personal beliefs so visibly and permanently
- Not wishing to appear different from other people
- Pressure from system managers to express particular values

Obviously, it is possible to lie about one's values whatever the circumstances and whatever the system. However, there are plenty of good reasons to be honest when using the VIDe system. For example:

- If required, the system can be set up so that users are anonymous (either entirely or at levels within the system)
- The system typically reveals a wide range of values per case. As a result it is very hard NOT to appear different from other people. Use of the system shows that even if people agree about what should be done, they tend to offer a cornucopia of perceptions and reasons why
- The system stands on the premise that there is no such thing as right and wrong values
- The reality of current health care practice (for example) is that there is already pressure on people to exhibit certain values rather than others. By revealing a plurality of values this sort of pressure becomes less tenable – if it remains once the system becomes commonly used, it will require a much deeper justification than 'this is normal practice', or 'this is what we do around here'
- By promoting Fulford's two-feet principle (p. 100 above) values-based transparency systems begin to change practice culture. As the culture changes to one which recognises values-pluralism, the idea that it is acceptable to impose one set of values only becomes increasingly suspect and open to challenge
- By means of a range of triggers set to alert the system administrator to significant conflicts between team members, the system works as a form of risk-management (and hostility reduction). In order for the risk-management function to work correctly, it is necessary for users to be honest. A further incentive to be honest is the prospect of one's decisions becoming part of a review of some kind, subject to detailed comparison and scrutiny

3. The values involved in decision-making are simply too complex to express

It may be that the fundamental reason why a particular decision was made is unknowable because human values tend to be so vague and manifold. For example, a doctor's decision to stop treating a patient may have a range of causes:

- Her feeling pressured on resources
- A personal judgement that the subject no longer really wants the treatment
- Her religious beliefs
- Personal experience of the type of pain the patient is experiencing
- Her level of interest in the patient
- Coercion from colleagues to make a particular decision
- Advice from friends
- Personal understanding of the law
- Clarity of communication between doctor and patient

Ultimately, which of these factors had which level of influence, may simply be too complex a matter ever to understand properly.

Nevertheless, using the VIDe system, tied electronically to patient record systems and broader data-warehoused records, it becomes possible to compare expressed reasons why decisions were made with actual outcomes. Potentially, this enables research into even the most complex relationships between values and actions.

4. Deceiving oneself

We are able to deceive ourselves in all sorts of ways. For example, in the case above it may be that the doctor was at some level aware that she was influenced by considerations of resource, but did not want to admit it to herself, and therefore did not give much weight to resources as she posted her analysis using the VIDe system.

There are two ways to deal with a problem such as this. The first is for the doctor in question to use the system in good faith, building up a portfolio of cases and reasons, and to attend training sessions in which she is encouraged to review her use of it. The second is for her to review other doctors' decisions and values reflectively. By doing so she will see a diversity of reasons recorded and may as a consequence feel more relaxed about revealing the evaluative basis for her decision-making.

Also:

- It might be that a doctor believes her values did not or could not enter into the deliberation because the evidence was decisive.

  In this case the doctor will simply be mistaken. If she inserts a random set of values into the system this will probably appear strange even in a single case, and will certainly appear strange when similar cases are compared: unless the doctor enters the same random data each time – which will also seem strange.
- It might be that the doctor believes she had no choice but to do what she did.

  This may be true, but if so this is all the more reason for the doctor to use the system to explain that although this is what she had to do her values were incompatible with this choice (or, if her values were compatible, to state that she was happy with the imposed choice).
- It might be that the doctor uses the system to find out what the most common response to this sort of proposal in these circumstances is, and decides merely to copy it.

  This may happen if the doctor (or any other user) exhibits an excessive need for conformity, to be part of the normal bulk of decision-making. If this is the case there is probably no way around it. However, it matters little so far as getting a good values-based picture, since the choice – I want to do what most other people do – is itself evaluative and expresses that doctor's desire to be part of the herd.

5. Sabotage

Crude attempts to sabotage the system – say by entering random data, or by expressing false values and reasons – are likely to be detected either at the coal-face (by people noticing that this is not the way the saboteur actually thinks) or when the saboteur's decision-making trends are audited either for him as an individual or in comparison with other people's trends.

More sophisticated attempts to sabotage the system – say by falsifying one's decision-making patterns subtly – ARE likely to succeed just as any other sophisticated attempts to deceive people are likely to succeed, at least for a time.

On the other hand, if people attempt sabotage, this in itself is a powerful endorsement of the system's worth. Something must be working for someone to want to stop it.

Do you allow people a free choice or do you select a limited range of options for them?

The Fulford approach allows people a free choice – they can explain any of their actions by appeal to any values. The VIDe approach limits the ways users can express their values by using set categories, meanings and questions. A casual observer might consider the former approach liberating and the latter overly restrictive. For example, she might object that the VIDe system:

- Restricts the meanings open to users
- Ties users' hands to only those values which can be said, written about and selected using a piece of software
- Forces users into significant compromises of meaning
- Limits users' reflective possibilities
- Makes values quantifiable when they are not
- Makes unique individually held values seem the same as everyone else's

However:

- It is possible to use the system to express most or all of the values necessary for professional decision-making (this is borne out by practical experience – no one objects that they cannot use the system to express what they want to).
- Different meanings can be included as appropriate
- The VIDe system actually expands reflective possibility by exposing us systematically to a range of considerations that might not have occurred to us (the meanings and questions contained in system); by exposing us instantly to other people's uses of the system, and their decisions and prejudices (through the reporting functions); by enabling shared and meaningful discussion as we review system use in context; by prompting us to challenge our own prejudices and to think in fresh ways (by seeing others' responses and through the feedback mechanisms built into the system).
- There is no reason why values should not be quantifiable, at least up to a point. The system is offered in the knowledge that it is foolish to count values as if they are bricks in a builder's yard – the human psyche is much more sophisticated than this. However, many values are easy to measure – for example choosing between 'I agree to carry out this person's wishes' and 'I do not agree to carry out this person's wishes'.
- Generally speaking our values are mostly, and perhaps entirely, common to us.

The VIDe system tries to enable people to reveal and see values using a shared language in a way they can feel comfortable with, but which renders their decision-making justifications comparable. An entirely free choice ends up leaving everything as it is, giving no more clarity that we have at present.

How you allow people to explain their values can affect the result you get

There is obviously a difference between the question:

> Do you think the USA should enter Iraq to free the people from the cruel dictator, Saddam Hussein?

and

> Do you think the USA should invade Iraq in order to secure oil supplies at a price affordable to US citizens?

As every questionnaire expert knows, the way and order in which questions are asked can have a profound influence on the answers. For example:

> "Do you think it should be possible for a pregnant woman to obtain a legal abortion if she is married and does not want any more children?" (Question A)

> "Do you think it should be possible for a pregnant woman to obtain a legal abortion if there is a strong chance of serious defect in the baby?" (Question B)

> In 1979, U-M researcher Howard Schuman asked these two questions as part of the Detroit Area Study, with half the 777 respondents asked in A-B order and half in B-A order. He found that support for abortion because a woman "does not want any more children" (A) was higher when this question was asked first and dropped dramatically when preceded by the child defect question (B). "This experiment has been repeated many times," notes psychologist Norbert Schwarz. "Although the absolute numbers vary, the pattern remains the same."[139]

And:

> How were the questions worded? The exact wording of survey questions can have a major influence on the results. Taking a close look at how the questions were worded is one of the most important things a reader can do to evaluate public opinion research. The order in which questions are asked can also affect a poll's results.

> Two types of questions frequently used in polls are 'forced choice' questions, where respondents are provided with a list of answers to choose from, and 'open-ended' questions, which allow respondents to give whatever answer they like. Open-ended questions are best used when the researchers know little about the public's opinions on a particular topic. The responses to an open-ended question reveal the entire range of beliefs people hold on the topic. The varied answers to open-ended questions are grouped into larger categories by the poll takers for reporting purposes. This must be done carefully to avoid biasing the conclusions.

> When asking questions about public policy issues such as education, forced choice questions work well when public opinion researchers already have some idea of the options the public is considering. Asking respondents to pick only one option from a list, or to rank the options, can reveal their priorities among alternatives in a way that an open-ended question cannot. What is included on the list of choices is crucial. The results only identify the public's priorities among the alternatives offered; if an option that has meaningful public support is left off, the results may be confusing or incomplete. In addition, the order in which the choices are presented must be systematically rotated during the polling to ensure unbiased results.[140]

The VIDe system uses both forced questions and opportunity for open-ended explanation. The original system has been designed with a deep understanding of the options and concerns of health professionals (later versions will work for other professionals and for the subjects of professional intervention). But it is inevitably biased. Most notably, in the current health care version respondents are asked to use understandings of health that are not universally held ('create autonomy', for instance).

However, the same is true for any system of eliciting values. Even just giving people a blank sheet of paper and asking them to write out what they think should be done about X or Y biases matters because:

- The question has been selected from other possible questions
- The answers given depend upon people's understandings of the evidence and its consequences, and these understandings can vary considerably
- The answers given depend upon people's general education, social standing, and personal experiences[141]

The VIDe version of **VDM** is all the stronger for recognising these realities.

CHAPTER FIVE

Goodbye Ethics Experts – The Democratic Promise of Values-Based Decision-Making

SUMMARY

- There is no such thing as an 'ethics expert'
- Transparent values-based decision-making is necessary where people in positions of authority claim to be making decisions in the interests of people subject to that authority, whether in private or public realms. It is also necessary where technical evidence and expertise is not decisive
- **VDM** will supersede ethics committees as traditionally conceived
- The role of ethics committees will evolve. Ethics committees will become co-ordinators of broad consultation about matters of pressing public concern, about the contexts in which these matters arise, and about **VDM** in general
- The enormous democratic potential of **VDM** is briefly outlined
- The truth is out there, Mr. Spock

———————— ◆ ————————

I am frequently approached by members of the news-media who invariably want to know what's ethical and unethical in topical situations. This is a typical communication:

Hi David,

Here are details of a debate from England. Can you help me please?

UK fertility body eases rules on embryo selection

By Alison Williams

LONDON, July 21 (Reuters) – Britain's fertility watchdog agreed on Wednesday to relax the rules governing clinics selecting embryos, to help parents find treatment for sick children by using cells from a baby brother or sister.

Critics say it will lead to the creation of so-called 'designer babies' where parents can choose image traits such as eye colour and will lead to many more discarded embryos.

But the Human Fertilisation and Embryology Authority (HFEA) said it took the decision for medical reasons to save the lives of sick siblings through matching tissue.

'I do not believe this is playing God. By definition you cannot play God,' Suzi Leather, chairman of the HFEA, told reporters.

David King, director of Human Genetics Alert pressure group, said: 'It is wrong to create a child simply as a means to an end, however good that end might be ... This violates the basic ethical principal that we should not use people as tools.'

Existing rules allowed fertility clinics to screen embryos for serious genetic disorders, but a number of recent cases have tested the legal boundaries and provoked a heated ethical debate on the merits of embryo selection.

Wednesday's decision will mean scientists can test embryos for a particular tissue type to harvest stem cells which could be transplanted to an ill child. Stem cells are master cells that can develop into specialised cells and be used to treat a range of illnesses.

The HFEA said each family would be considered on a case by case basis when the treatment was proven to be a last resort ...

REUTERS

Reut 17:59 07-21-04

We would basically like some comment about the ethical argument – is it ethical in light of the fact it will help sick children?

The critics I have spoken to are predominantly concerned with the small steps being taken which they claim are slowly leading towards designer babies and general human cloning. Is there a line which can be drawn?

Any enlightenment will be much appreciated.

Thanks,

Virginia Jones
Newstalk JB Journalist
Newsroom: 09 4733255

Here's my reply:

Hi Virginia

The thing is that there are no 'ethical rules' in this area. No one can answer the question 'is this ethical?' with real authority – as no doubt you've found out. There are only opinions and hopes and fears – and we would be wise to recognise that this is basically what's going on.

How you feel about this depends in large part on what you think an embryo is – and that is a value judgement: David King uses the word 'child' to describe the embryo and the pejorative word 'tool' to imply that this isn't what children should be. But people on the other side see only unconscious cells that might be used to help actual children. There is no way these guys are ever going to agree.

For my part, given that IVF usually produces more viable embryos than can ever be born, and given that these embryos are routinely destroyed, and given that naturally millions of embryos are unviable every year, I favour using science on them to help sick children. I don't think this is the same as or bound to lead to designer babies. Equally I don't see that designer babies are such a bad thing either . . . But that's another argument.

Hope this helps.

David

David Seedhouse

What else could I honestly say? What else can anyone honestly say? The only alternative approach is to claim or imply privileged knowledge of some ethical truth. Perhaps like this:

Hi Virginia

Clearly David King is correct in his views. As a Professor of Ethics I endorse what he says and would also say that the HFEA are clearly in breach of the basic ethical principle of the right to life/beneficence/non-maleficence/thou shalt not kill/ . . . (Virginia, you can quote me as asserting as many of these as you like).

The fact that sick children might be helped is not relevant here. There are other, moral ways to help sick children.

As every right-thinking person knows, we must respect God's will and intentions in these matters.

Yours truly,

Ethics Professor, BA (Hons), PhD

Or perhaps like this:

Hi Virginia

Clearly the HFEA is correct in its view. As a Professor of Ethics I endorse what this eminent body says and would also say that the David King and his colleagues are clearly in breach of the basic ethical principle of the right to life (of the sick children)/beneficence/non-maleficence/thou shalt not kill/ . . . (Virginia, you can quote me as asserting as many of these as you like).

The fact that sick children might be helped is crucial here. Using unwanted embryos is a perfectly moral and efficient way to help sick children.

We must be rational and realistic in these matters.

Yours truly,

Ethics Professor, BA (Hons), PhD

For most of my career I have been tagged an ethics expert. Yet no one can be an ethics expert if being an ethics expert means knowing for certain how to live right. I may sometimes be able to help people structure their thinking better than they could without me, and I am well placed to explain a practical philosophical approach to health work.[81] But neither I nor anyone else has privileged access to moral truth.

Nevertheless, thousands of inflexible ethical pronouncements are made daily by ethics experts and ethics committees, blustering under the impression that they have the authority to decree ethical standards for everyone else.[142,143]

There will always be a need for people who can explain the evidence associated with social affairs, and for people with experience in debating them (very occasionally I find I can reveal an aspect to a situation which less experienced participants have not noticed). However, the need for knowledge and experience should not be confused with a need for mythical experts in value-judgement.

This is demonstrated by every use of VIDe software. Here, for example, is an obstetrics and gynaecology case (posted under for urgent response by an obstetrician on the **Values Exchange**® – patient and participant's names changed):

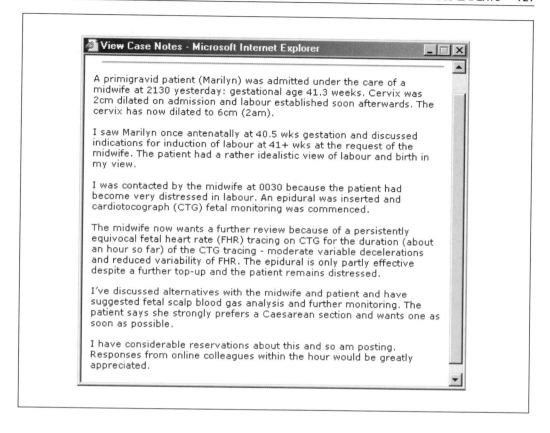

A primigravid patient (Marilyn) was admitted under the care of a midwife at 2130 yesterday: gestational age 41.3 weeks. Cervix was 2cm dilated on admission and labour established soon afterwards. The cervix has now dilated to 6cm (2am).

I saw Marilyn once antenatally at 40.5 wks gestation and discussed indications for induction of labour at 41+ wks at the request of the midwife. The patient had a rather idealistic view of labour and birth in my view.

I was contacted by the midwife at 0030 because the patient had become very distressed in labour. An epidural was inserted and cardiotocograph (CTG) fetal monitoring was commenced.

The midwife now wants a further review because of a persistently equivocal fetal heart rate (FHR) tracing on CTG for the duration (about an hour so far) of the CTG tracing - moderate variable decelerations and reduced variability of FHR. The epidural is only partly effective despite a further top-up and the patient remains distressed.

I've discussed alternatives with the midwife and patient and have suggested fetal scalp blood gas analysis and further monitoring. The patient says she strongly prefers a Caesarean section and wants one as soon as possible.

I have considerable reservations about this and so am posting. Responses from online colleagues within the hour would be greatly appreciated.

Clearly there is room for expertise in this case. Experience in and knowledge of obstetrics is necessary, and some knowledge of psychology and relevant legal and ethical analysis would be very helpful. And yet, however many similar cases you've been involved in, an ocean of VALUES-RAW choices remains. For example:

- Do you agree or disagree?
- Who is most important in this case? Marilyn? The baby? A broader group of people? Are they equally important?
- How emotionally comfortable with the proposal (that the patient's request should be accepted) are you?
- What do you think the chief risk is?
- Would you personally be willing to perform the operation?
- Is communication distorted? If it is, is it distorted to such an extent that Marilyn's value-judgement has also been distorted? Is it possible to distort a value-judgement? Do people have normal value sets, or do our values fluctuate according to circumstance?
- If someone is appointed to advocate for the baby, what values should she advocate?

Figures 42 to **46** show how real obstetricians dealt with this case (all images © VIDe Ltd).

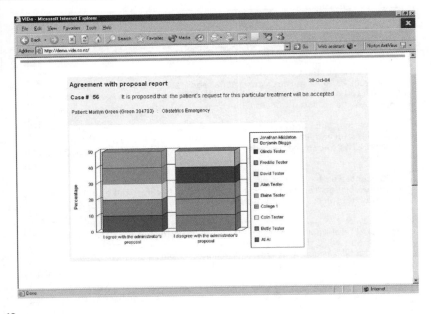

Figure 42

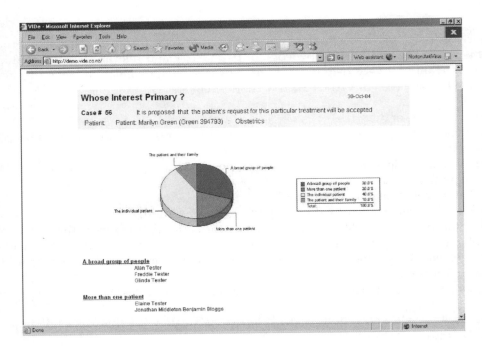

Figure 43

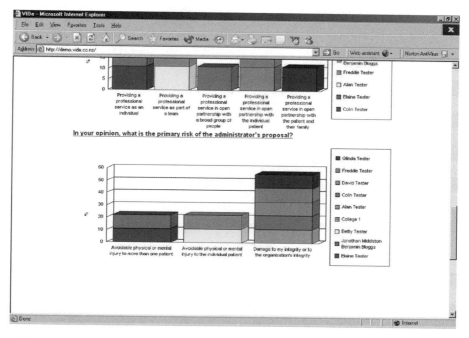

Figure 44

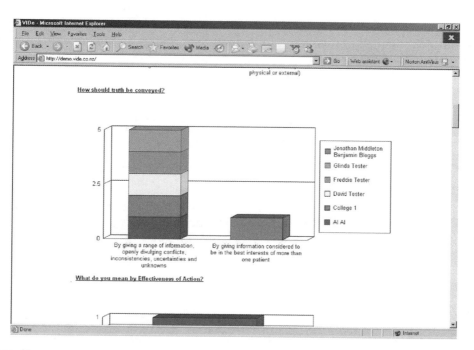

Figure 45

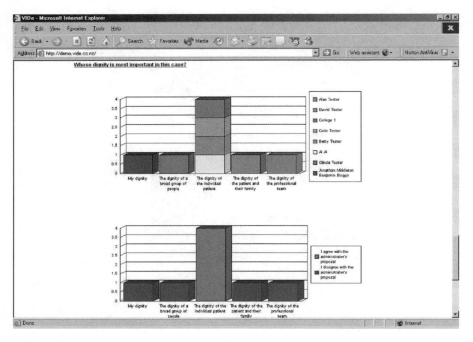

Figure 46

This range of views and attitudes is utterly typical of the use of **VDM** software. Either there is a truly moral answer to each and every problem posted, and some or all participants get it wrong every time, or there is never a right answer and all participants make sincere attempts to discover and explain their values, in the hope of a reaching a transparent, human solution.

THE NECESSITY OF TRANSPARENT VALUES-BASED DECISION-MAKING

Transparent values-based decision-making is necessary in the following circumstances:

- Where people in positions of authority claim to be making decisions in the interests of people subject to that authority, whether in private or public realms
- Where technical evidence and expertise is not decisive

WHAT IF....?

Now that it is possible to reveal values systematically and meaningfully over large numbers of people the possibilities for social improvement are staggering.

WHAT IF VDM WERE USED TO REPLACE ETHICS COMMITTEES?

Are there any reasons that should compel us to keep ethics committees in their present form? Typical arguments in favour of ethics committees are that they:

- Ensure ethical behaviour and research
- Include a wide range of opinion and ensure that every case is fully explored by people with a range of viewpoints
- Are objective and impartial
- Are consistent[144]
- Bring technical expertise in addition to ethical expertise
- Gain and provide experience in deliberating on ethical matters
- Record deliberations for open scrutiny
- Prevent powerful people doing whatever they want[145]
- Are a filtering mechanism when there are more proposals than can be financed
- Give invaluable feedback to researchers

ARE THESE REASONS GOOD ENOUGH?

Let's consider each of these reasons in turn.

Ethics committees ensure ethical behaviour and research

The nature of ethical behaviour and research is forever open to debate. Consequently, it should be no surprise at all that different ethics committees regularly come to different conclusions about the same issues,[146] and the same ethics committees at different times reach different conclusions about exactly the same cases.[144]

Furthermore, ethics committees can scrutinise and decide only between those proposals that pass before them. They have little or no brief to consider the context of the proposals, and no power to alter their context even if they want to. For example, an ethics committee might scrutinise a set of proposals, each sponsored by a drug company, to undertake research on a particular type of psychiatric medication, where there is only enough money to fund 50 per cent of the proposals. Their task: to approve the most ethical 50 per cent. However, the ethics committee members can do nothing to question whether this sort of research should be pursed *per se*, or whether there might be better uses of research funding.

Ethics committees include a wide range of opinion and ensure that every case is fully explored by people with a range of viewpoints

This might be true of some ethics committees. However, for some it is certainly false. For example:

Possible Conflict of Interest Among Committee Members

The situation regarding the safety of the meningitis program was further called into question in September, when it was learned that four of the medical experts responsible for advising the government on the meningitis vaccine's safety had financial ties to one or more of the vaccine's manufacturers.

Professor Janet Barbyshire, a member of the Committee on Safety of Medicines and director of the Medical Research Council, was found to have received support for academic research from Wyeth and Chiron, the makers of the Meningitec and Meninjugate vaccines currently used in the U.K.

In addition, three members of the government's Joint Committee on Vaccination and Immunisation were shown to have declared interests in vaccine manufacturers. One member, Dr. David Goldblatt of the Institute of Child Health, was found to have served on an advisory panel for Wyeth and to have received research grants from both Wyeth and North American Vaccines, which produces a third meningitis vaccine (Neisvac). Another, Professor Keith Cartwright, received funding to 'evaluate candidate meningicoccal vaccines' for use in the United Kingdom.

'This is a question of propriety,' said Norman Baker, the Liberal Democrat party's consumer affairs spokesman, who has tabled parliamentary questions about the financial interests of the committee members. 'There must be enough independent people around to give advice without turning to those who clearly have a conflict of interests. I am not questioning their academic credentials, but with the best will in the world, their judgments must be looked at in that context.'[147]

Certainly, if an ethics committee is drawn from a wide range of backgrounds there is more chance of it including a wide range of opinion. However, ethics committees tend to attract people with very strong views about moral rights and wrongs, and almost inevitably particular outlooks come to dominate. Furthermore:

- Groups that meet regularly tend to form predictable thinking trends and even 'group think'
- Every committee meets within a cultural context. For example, within a hospital, in a Health Authority, within a certain country, in a certain era, and so on.
- Every committee creates a cultural context. For example, once it has become established that every proposal should be scrutinised to ensure, say, informed consent and the protection of vulnerable groups then these things tend to become the focus of attention – they tend to become considered to be THE ethical priorities even though there is an indefinite number of ethical questions that might be raised. In turn this means that other issues receive less attention – indigenous people's interests, for example (see pp. 86–87 above)

Ethics committees are objective and impartial

It depends what is meant by 'objective'. If the phrase is intended to mean 'ethics committees establish what is truly ethical, independent of human opinion' then it is plainly false. It is also false if it is supposed to mean that ethics committees establish their recommendations dispassionately (no real world deliberation can ACTUALLY commit Spock's Mistake).

However, if the phrase is supposed to mean 'ethics committees are not entirely subjective', then it is plausible. But it isn't a very big or very remarkable claim. It merely says that ethics committees deliberate in order to reach conclusions beyond the views of a single subject.

Ethics committees are consistent

Ethics committees may or may not be consistent. Whatever the case, it is important to remember that consistency is not necessarily a good thing – bad judgements can be made just as consistently as good ones.

Ethics committees do tend to be consistent in a general sense. That is, they operate within a tight, culturally insulated rational field – a manufactured rational field in which they are meant to uphold vague standards like beneficence, non-maleficence, respect autonomy and justice.[148] And where they are certainly NOT meant to criticise or change either these standards or the prevailing social circumstances which create and sponsor the committees themselves.

Ethics committees bring technical expertise in addition to ethical expertise

Ethics committees gain and provide experience in deliberating on ethical matters

There is no doubt that these things are usually true.

Ethics committees record deliberations for open scrutiny

This may or may not be true, dependent on the committee's terms of reference. It is rarely true of in-house hospital or university research ethics committees. Their pronouncements may sometimes become public knowledge, but not their deliberations and internal debates and disagreements.[145]

Ethics committees prevent powerful people doing whatever they want

Clearly this is not true. There are laws most of us obey most of the time, there are peer pressures, and there are social values and mores. These mediators of ego are much more powerful than ethics committees.

Even more to the point, it is common knowledge that even where there are ethics committees people very often do what they want to anyway.[149]

Ethics committees are filtering mechanisms when there are more proposals than can be financed

Ethics committees give invaluable feedback to researchers

There is no doubting these points either. Equally there is no reason why proposals have to be filtered as they are at the moment. And technical feedback can be given through all manner of mechanisms; as can legal, professional or any other sort of feedback. In fact there is nothing ethics committees can sensibly do that cannot be done better without resort to ethics committees. If we were to establish a way to involve everyone in social decision-making (or at least a wide range of representative groups) much would change for the better. For example, involving indigenous people in fair proportion would open up external pressure on Western ethics committees' rational fields by emphasising justice, respect for the environment, group involvement and debate as being at least as important as individual consent.

If ethics committees were to take nothing for granted, all sorts of cherished Western ethical ideals might be challenged: and since ethics committees are not legislative bodies, why should they take anything for granted? Perhaps it would turn out – against received wisdom – that people are happy to be part of research projects without their explicit consent so long as the projects are clearly for the public good. Perhaps we would find that some people are prepared NOT to be treated if a younger or more deserving person can be treated in their stead. Or perhaps we would discover that most people feel it is better if information is withheld from seriously ailing patients. Who knows?

What is certain is that the:

> ...currently dominant quasi-legal form of clinical bioethics (which) prescribes good outcomes in the form of increasingly complex ethical rules and regulations...[135]

would come to be seen for what it is: pseudo-law, typically enforcing a limited range of white middle-class prejudices and (almost certainly) a minority view of what is in the public interest.

THE FUTURE OF ETHICS COMMITTEES AFTER VDM

It is unlikely that even very widespread use of **VDM** will herald the end of ethics committees. Nevertheless, as more and more of us who are not part of ethics committees become used to having our values heard and recorded, it is inevitable that ethics committees' functions will evolve.

Ethics committees will be called upon to make fewer expert ethical judgements (ultimately they won't be invited to make any). However, they will very likely still be asked to:

- Collate evidence in order to inform potentially controversial decisions
- Organise questions and discussion about these decisions
- Set out possible options for dealing with these decisions
- (Possibly) express a collective view about these decisions

But they will not do this within their committee walls, as they almost always do at the moment. Rather, in addition to the above tasks, ethics committees of the future will:

- Educate citizens about evidence, values and the use of **VDM**
- Present specific evidence in a form accessible to citizens who are not expert in the subject matter of potentially controversial decisions
- Administer **VDM** systems in order to enable non-committee members to express their feelings and outline their reasoning about potentially controversial decisions
- Co-ordinate citizens' use of **VDM** systems
- Present the results of applied **VDM** on a public website, for all to see
- Research the general public's values and values-trends
- Display the results of their growing research on a public website, for all to see
- Work with other ethics committees in a network of open debate, research and education about VDM

WHAT IF....

VDM were to be used routinely for major local authority decisions (in-fill housing? new shopping centres? traffic controls? leisure facilities? pest control and the use of insecticides? fluoridation? vaccination? product advertising? the content of children's television? the level of violence permitted in readily available films?). Every member of the population able to use a PC could regularly contribute to such decision-making, and a growing store of values-trends could be kept and applied to help formulate further questions.

Some local councils already appreciate the importance of this, but do not as yet have the means of achieving it:

February 2002

THE BENEFITS OF VALUE-BASED DECISION-MAKING: A DISCUSSION AMONG CITY OFFICIALS

---

by JoAnne Speers

At the League's 2001 Executive Forum in Monterey, a standing-room-only crowd of city officials gathered to discuss the ethical principles of decision-making in city service.

The discussion centered on a hypothetical scenario involving a proposal to use the city's power of eminent domain. In this scenario, a city was considering acquiring property from private landowners to allow a large business to locate in the city. Various council members also had personal relationships with individuals whose interests would be affected both positively and negatively by the city's decision.

The law can define the minimum of ethical action, but not the height of ethical conduct.

In discussing the issues presented by the scenario, at least five core principles emerged as ethical issues for local officials to consider:

- **Whole Community.** Which decision advances the good of the whole community? Which decision does more harm than good?
- **Individual Rights.** Is the decision respectful of individuals' rights and interests? Is the decision fair?
- **Process.** Has the decision-making process been open to community input and feedback? Do members of the public feel satisfied that their opinions have been heard and considered by decision makers?
- **Legality.** Have all relevant legal considerations been identified and satisfied?
- **Alternatives.** Would other approaches or modifications to the proposal before the council involve fewer trade-offs?

Public service is about acting in the interest of the larger community.

Needless to say, applying these principles can be difficult. At least two of the principles can be inherently contradictory: For example, decisions that benefit the whole community can harm individuals' interests. Weighing these competing considerations is part of the challenge of local leadership . . .

Being honest in your capacity as a council member can influence how others perceive your integrity.

The panelists generally agreed that it would be unethical for a public agency to confer a benefit on an individual that would be detrimental to the community as a whole. Thus the friendships, personal interests and business relationships that might otherwise influence an individual's decisions in private life must not influence a public official's decision. For example, in the City of Santa Clara's code of ethics and values city officials agreed that the goal is to make 'impartial decisions, free of bribes, unlawful gifts, narrow political interests and financial or other personal interests that impair [our] independence of judgment or action.' . . . .

Many people are intimidated by the formality of council meetings and don't want to talk.

The Open Process

The panelists voiced strong, unanimous agreement about the importance of an *open process* in achieving ethical decision-making . . .

Unfortunately, there is no right or wrong way to strike a balance.

Margaret Finlay, council member of Duarte and a League board member, asked whether there is ever a good time or a good reason for council members to meet privately with developers, without staff or others present. The consensus rapidly expressed by the panel and others was no. This inadvisable practice is antithetical to the open process that builds public confidence in local officials' ability to put the community's interests first when making decisions. . . . . . .

What Are Your Thoughts?

One of the objectives of the Executive Forum discussion was to collaborate on a framework for identifying and analyzing potential ethical dilemmas. This is the first installment of an ongoing dialogue about these issues. The Institute for Local Self Government (ILSG), as the League's nonprofit research arm and session sponsor, is interested in collecting additional perspectives from local officials on this issue. Should local officials take the initiative on having such conversations? If so, are there ways of explaining a decision that seem to avoid or minimize the unpleasantness that can occur when a local official tells a supporter that the official sees the issue differently?

To share your views and experiences with ethics issues, please log on to ILSG's website www.ilsg.org/publicconfidence.[150]

Imagine how helpful **VDM** would be in facilitating the processes described in the article boxed above. Undoubtedly the council's desire for open process could be simply and dramatically achieved.

What if...

VDM were to be used in prisons, by both prisoners and guards?

What if all concerned could post their views on any proposal of mutual interest? At the very least there would be increased communication, and possibly increased understanding, between inmates and prison officers.

What if...

VDM were to be used in schools by pupils and teachers in order to debate curriculum development or uniforms, or tattoos, or food menus, or discipline: do the students value the same goals and strategies as the teachers, and if not what are the implications? Given the obvious imbalance in power within schools, it would be fascinating to see what insights would be produced by the anonymous use of the software.

What if...

VDM were to be used by magistrates as a learning tool? It is well-known that magistrates in different areas[151,152] apply different sentences for the same offences. It is difficult to imagine what factors other than values can explain this. If this were to be proven through the use of **VDM** software, a brand new set of policy choices would emerge for the governance of magistrates.

What if...

VDM were to be used by local and central government, directly, for key decisions? The software could be used to facilitate simple referenda, but could also be used in more subtle ways either to detect values-trends amongst the population, or to explain the preferences and reasoning processes of government policy-makers themselves. Policy-makers could use the software – using their real names and giving their real feelings and reasoning – and their deliberations could be made publicly available as reports on the **Values Exchange**® website.

Of course, there would still be disagreements – 'we don't want the airport in our backyard', 'we don't want the airport in OUR backyard either', 'actually, we policy-makers think you SHOULD have the airport in your backyard' – but at least the values-base of any disagreement would be clear to everyone.

What if...

VDM were to be used in the legal system? What if judges were able to explain their decisions by openly expressing their values in addition to the traditional factors? Judges repeatedly make value-judgements,[153,154] why not own up to the fact? Why not make a virtue of it? Why not research and display these values for everyone to see? What if jurors could do this? What if **VDM** systems were made a part of jury deliberations? What if, in addition to assessing the evidence, jurors could explain their prejudices and their reasoning, and what if these could be displayed instantly to them? What if the jurors knew that these would be made public knowledge (with appropriate protections)? Wouldn't this be more honest and more likely to ensure justice? It would, at least, ensure that justice would be seen to be done.[155]

What if...

VDM were used routinely by government grant awarding bodies in their deliberations over which research or which commercial enterprises to support? What if such use were mandatory on public officials, and what if there were methods in place to compare different bodies' deliberations? And what if these reports were open to public scrutiny? What value-judgements went into awarding Professor Smith $1 million while declining Professor Jones' application? In some cases technical matters will be in play, but (as everyone knows) very often this type of decision is to do with relationships, politics, personal judgements about the desirability of the research, balancing financial priorities and so on. Once the public could see what any honest research grant committee member recognises at her very first meeting, the question: 'why aren't OUR values equally valued?' would be unavoidable. More than that, we might begin to ask: given that every research project is based on values, and given that there is an infinite number of research goals in the world, why are we restricted only to a very small, usually scientific-establishment sponsored set of projects? Instead of research into X and Y, why can't we fund research into the redistribution of wealth? Why can't we fund research into complementary therapies at the same level as research into conventional drug therapies? What about researching ways of achieving cultural harmony, alternatives to petrol-driven transport, reform of the school system, research into the causes of warfare, research into how to prevent warfare? Why not fund these on equal terms with state sponsorship of the arms industry?

Once you reveal values and their social influence you lay bare an ocean of possibility.

What if...

VDM were to be used by 'intelligence gathering services' to help explain why they regard some evidence as reliable and other evidence as unreliable (judgements about the reliability of evidence sooner or later rest on values)? What if VDM were to be used to discover why intelligence services seek a particular sort of evidence and disregard other evidence altogether? What if VDM were used to try to explain intelligence services' level of confidence in their evidence? Evidence collected by intelligence services about the presence and threat of weapons of mass destruction in Iraq was found to be utterly wrong.[156] If we could at least SEE the values background to the collection and interpretation of the evidence in such cases we could form a more balanced and realistic view of its accuracy, and be able to judge how seriously we should heed it.

What if...

VDM were to be used routinely to bring victims and perpetrators of crime together? What if the results of these shared deliberations were publicised widely – for example, in schools and other youth environments?

What if...

VDM were to be used for arbitration and for finding the common values-basis to all disputes? In every case there will ALWAYS be considerable common ground because human beings share so many rational fields, as we saw in **Chapter 3**. Although some of the rational fields that make up the larger rational fields of, say, fundamentalist Islam and Hugh Hefner will be incommensurable, there will always be many points of contact: love, desire, sense of belonging, sense of cause, kindness and cruelty, for example.

What if...

VDM were to be used to settle disputes between nations? What if **VDM** were to be used according to international law before nations could go to war with each other?

What if...

VDM were to be used to settle disputes between religious groups? Wouldn't one expect more commonality than difference in such cases?

What if...

VDM were to be used to show the futility of much 'ethical debate' about abortion and euthanasia? For example to prove the obvious: that such discussion simply relies upon different and conflicting assumptions about what is valuable? And what if we could move forward from this point of futility to find common ground to build on? It surely exists. Whatever side they're on, the protagonists undoubtedly agree that human life is valuable – might it not be possible to use a range of case studies to help all concerned draw a more harmonious line around the limits of what counts as a good life?

What if...

There were a **Values Exchange** available to everyone – values-exchange.com?

VALUES-BASED DECISION-MAKING AS A THERAPEUTIC TOOL

There is increasing evidence that the more choice patients have in their health care, the better the outcomes. Typically, research in this area has focused on the effects of permitting patients to administer their own pain relief, rather than receiving it at the convenience of health staff; the level of motivation patients have to undertake therapy; and involving patients in decision-making about smoking, alcohol and diabetes care.[157-166]

The basis of this research and practice to support autonomy as therapy is firmly rooted in values-based decision-making. Not only does the work explicitly value autonomy (i.e. value it as a good thing in principle that patients should have as much control as possible over what happens to them), but by valuing autonomy it automatically opens the door for diverse values and priorities to come into play. Since patients do not all have the same attitudes and aspirations, emphasising their autonomy is also to emphasise diversity. Some patients want as much control as possible, others are happier to take advice. Some patients want maximum pain relief, others want to be as alert as possible to experience life and to interact with others. Some patients want medication or surgery, others prefer non-invasive interventions.

Values-based decision-making as explicit therapy moves **VDM** to its logical conclusion. Since values are the root of conscious autonomy/conscious choices, if we want to support autonomy as fully as possible (which we should if we wish to create the greatest degree of health possible[81]) we should enable patients to make the most explicit value judgements they possibly can. This might be achieved by using the **VDM** software to ascertain what they value most, by:

- Using vignettes about what might happen to them
- Providing a specific list of goals and outcomes to choose from
- Providing an open choice about what they might realistically hope to achieve, given their circumstances
- Showing them what other patients in similar circumstances have valued
- Showing them what health professionals think they should value
- Comparing patient priorities against health professional priorities
- Devising ways for patients to use the same software systems as professionals in order to judge levels of consensus and conflict.

VALUES-BASED DECISION-MAKING AS A RESEARCH TOOL

Once **VDM** is established as a therapeutic tool, it will be a relatively short step to using values-based software systems for research into the relationship between value-judgements (of either the professional or the patient or both) and actual outcomes. Because decisions are composed of preferences and reasoning, we might hypothesise along the following lines:

- The values and reasoning of health professionals have an effect on the success of health care interventions
- The values and reasoning of patients have an effect on the success of health care interventions
- The greater the disharmony between health professional and patient values the less successful health care interventions are

These are highly generalised hypotheses, which would have to be distilled into specific research projects. But there is no reason, so long as we can detect values in a plausible and consistent way, why such research projects should not be undertaken.

For example, one might convert the general hypothesis to:

- In cases of first time involuntary detention for the diagnosis of schizophrenia in female patients aged 30–35, the greater the disharmony between health professional and patient values the longer the period between admission and discharge

Or

- In paediatric treatment for condition X, the greater the disharmony between health professional and child patient values, the less successful therapy for condition X is

It may be that extensive research finds no relationship at all, forcing the unlikely conclusion that human interactions and relationships are immaterial in health care (such a conclusion would fly in the face of considerable research on stress, mind-body effects, and the importance of caring – to name but three values-based concepts).[137] And if research began to show that there is indeed a relationship between values and physical outcomes, imagine what an impact this would have on the education, selection and retention of health professionals.

WHAT WE CAN HOPE FOR

It is beyond dispute that once a decision-maker has a clear picture of his values, and of how these relate to his decision-making, he will become more insightful and therefore almost certainly a more rounded decision-maker. Furthermore, once he better understands his colleagues' reasoning processes and motivations, he is very likely to work more effectively and openly with them: agreements will be acknowledged as such, and disagreements will continually be open to informed inspection and debate.

It is also beyond dispute that patients will expect greater consistency of decision-making from professionals, because they will have access to reasoning and justification processes that previously were mostly or entirely hidden from them. There is also the realistic potential for patients to become FULLY involved, as equals, in all the values-based aspects of medical decision-making processes. It is worth emphasising this point one final time: while it is obviously impossible for anyone to be expert in more than a handful of technical matters, and as a rule therefore sensible for those who are not technically expert to follow expert advice, it is NOT POSSIBLE for anyone to be more expert than anyone else in matters of value. Values are preferences – every waking person has preferences and can almost always express them in some way. Of course it can be said (and frequently is said) that people's preferences are unwise or misguided, but this judgement too is nothing more than a matter of preference (unless there is some evidence that the person in question is unaware of, or cannot adequately comprehend). Essentially we judge and react to most human situations as equals, however young or old, clever or not clever we are.

VDM guarantees the equal involvement of all interested parties in a non-technical system that acts to render explicit UNIVERSAL tendencies of human life. What's more, these tendencies are turned into evidence: there can no longer be simple-minded resort to 'common sense' or 'most people would agree' or 'the evidence tells us what to do' or 'we know best' or 'do as you're told' because these expressions will be seen for what they are: crude gestures that say nothing more than 'my values are better than your values, so there...'.

TEN REASONS WHY WE NEED VDM

1. IT MEANS WE CAN TURN OUR VALUES INTO EVIDENCE   By using **VDM** we can see and understand our values and the values of others in context – our values can become concrete evidence to help us see how and why we make the decisions we do

2. VALUES ARE FIRST, EVIDENCE IS SECOND   By using **VDM** we can understand the extent to which our values affect our decisions – we can learn to appreciate that our values influence everything we do

3. DIFFERENT LEVELS OF TECHNICAL EXPERTISE DO NOT IMPLY DIFFERENT LEVELS OF EXPERTISE IN VALUING   By using **VDM** we can understand that while there are many differences in human technical expertise, we are all equally able to value and we are all equally instinctive

4. APPRECIATION OF DIFFERENCE   By using **VDM** we can appreciate that our values and instincts (and the ways these affect our reasoning) can vary considerably between individuals

5. EMOTION AND REASON ARE ONE   By using **VDM** we will never forget that our values require logic and our logic requires values if we are to act in the social world

6. REALISM ABOUT ETHICS   By using **VDM** we can see that ethical analysis is a matter of reflecting on evidence and values, with the genuine intent of finding the most reasonable solution to our problems – ethics is not dictatorial, there are no answers that are TRULY ethical

7. THERAPEUTIC POSSIBILITY   By using **VDM** we can learn to take patients seriously by recognising the diversity of their values, and the possible effect these values might have on prescribed therapies

8. RESEARCH   By using **VDM** we can begin to research the effects of values on clinical outcomes

9. GOODBYE ETHICS EXPERTS   By using **VDM** we can make paternalistic, 'expert' ethics committees and individual 'ethics experts' redundant, once and for all

10. TOLERANCE   Most important of all, by using **VDM** we will realise that if the evaluative/instinctive/classified/environmental SOURCE of rational fields is transparent then every rational field is potentially explicable: transparency and explicability create the possibility of tolerance.

There is a world of possibility waiting.

THE TRUTH IS OUT THERE, MR. SPOCK...

SPOCK: Emotional, isn't she?

SAREK: She has always been so.

SPOCK: Indeed. Why did you marry her?'

SAREK: It seemed the logical thing to do at the time.

Sarek is Spock's father. They are discussing Spock's mother.[167]

Epilogue

Though I have been interested in rationality since I was a university student, it is only now that I am gaining a USEFUL understanding of it.

Twenty years ago, in my PhD thesis, I argued against the 'rationalist' view that:

> ...'passion' can be relegated to a minor position...[168]

and (vaguely) advocated:

> ...a more tolerant and balanced philosophy instead.[168]

The foundation of my argument was that because definition requires consistency, and rationality is made up of inconsistent elements (logic and passion), rationality cannot be defined. Whenever anyone tries, something crucial is inevitably lost.

For example, consider this typical definition of rationality:

> n 1: the state of having good sense and sound judgment; 'his rationality may have been impaired'; 'he had to rely less on reason than on rousing their emotions' [syn: *reason, reasonableness*] 2: the quality of being consistent with or based on logic [syn: *rationalness*][169]

And this standard definition of rationalism:

> (rationalism is) the belief or principle that actions and opinions should be based on reason rather than on emotion or religion[170]

Not only do both definitions exclude emotion, they cast reason directly AGAINST it. But if human rationality consists of BOTH logic and emotion (as it obviously does) definitions like these are bound to distort our view of it.

Troubled by how much we were overlooking, I came to the conclusion that we should think of rationality as a concept, since concepts are able to accommodate personal perceptions and ambiguities which definitions cannot:

> ...(the concept of rationality) is like an abstract picture which includes many disparate and seemingly incompatible elements which nevertheless can be meaningful if seen together... it is crucially important that this picture is seen to *remain abstract*; if it becomes clear or 'realistic' then this is a false clarity, a clarity which, ironically, obscures the concept of rationality. To adopt a *'definition'* of rationality is to encourage this false clarity.[171]

I was convinced that rationality is the central human ideal; I knew it was a serious mistake to try to define it, and I was very taken by a hazy idea that we should understand it as a perpetually evolving, non-figurative painting:

> I intend this metaphor to conjure up an image of a picture which has unlikely, uncon-nected, and seemingly incompatible shapes, colours, and textures; but which is neverthe-less a *whole* picture – an inconsistent whole, a living whole to which the artist ('culture', 'society', groups of human beings, or individual human beings) can add or subtract. Cru-cially, this addition or subtraction should be done only in such a way as *to preserve the abstractness of the picture* . . . the abstract picture is able, because of its nature, to contain the various elements and manifestations of the split, and to contain them in a moral way – in such a way as ultimately to serve the general interest of humanity. **The various elements of the abstract picture, when taken together, can go to make up a frame for the picture; and this frame, in turn, can hold the picture together**. If certain of these elements are not thought important (for instance those elements from the 'human' side of the split), and so are removed from the frame, then the abstract picture can become unbalanced and may *appear* to be clear or 'realistic'. But this is a false, 'defined', clarity which can obscure the true nature of the picture. The concept of rationality can, because of its 'framed abstract-ness', act as a guide to human reasoning, and hence to human action.

> An awareness of the concept of rationality can impress upon human beings that a civilised and moral attitude depends on the seemingly incompatible manifestations of the split constantly being seen together. To take just one manifestation of the split as an example: an awareness of rationality can emphasise the importance of the assertion that neither 'logical rules' and 'scientific principles', nor 'human emotion' and 'passion' should be recognised exclusively when decisions are being made in the world.   [bold added][172]

I'm sure I didn't fully understand what I was trying to say when I wrote these paragraphs in 1984. I knew I was onto something important, but I hadn't grasped it properly. I certainly couldn't explain it to anyone else.

I was struggling to come up with a device which could include logic and passion in balance, with constructive, humane implications. The best I could do at the time was to liken rationality to an abstract picture framed by elements of the picture itself (see the sentence in bold in the quote above). But of course even the most abstract picture cannot be the same as its frame. There is either a picture AND a frame, or there is a picture without a frame, or there is a frame without a picture.

With hindsight it is stunningly obvious that all I had to do to express myself clearly was to say that the frame and the picture are different, but intimately and necessarily related: technical reason needs to be framed to make sense, emotional reason has to become logical if it is to have any constructive impact on the world at large.

UNDERSTANDING AND MISUNDERSTANDING

Thinking of rationality like this helps explain why human beings so often misunderstand each other (seeing rational fields in isolation from their frames is guaranteed to mislead).

Of course, it is easy enough NOT to be deceived when we see DISTINCTLY conflicting rational fields. If, for example, we view the goals and strategies of a warmongering general and a peace protestor side by side we don't really NEED to see the frames to know that very different attitudes and circumstances have created their respective rational fields. It is also instantly apparent that the 'blunt surgeon' I describe at page xv of this book forms his actions according to different values from mine. How-ever, most social situations are more subtle than this, and this is where confusion comes.

It is exceedingly common for it to appear to us that we are on the same wavelength as other people when we are not, because our frames are significantly different but we don't see it. We are naturally inclined to want to be in sympathy with others, yet we would be better advised to look out for differences in frames rather than take reassurance solely from more temporary behaviour patterns (ask any marriage guidance counsellor).

AN EXAMPLE

I used to puzzle about why I keep hitting brick walls when trying to communicate my ideas about health to people within the medical system. For the most part we seem to understand each other perfectly well, but when we talk about 'health goals' or 'health gain' we instantly lose contact.

It is obvious now that we misunderstand each other because we don't share frames, even though we frequently have the same goals and strategies (the same applies to my communications with establishment bioethicists). Different frames can create both harmonious AND conflicting rational fields. By noticing only the similar ones, and by using the same terms (for example 'health' or 'ethics'), we are lulled into a false sense of accord. Yes we agree about a lot of things, but fundamentally we misunderstand each other because we are blind to the frames which create and bind our pictures.

I think health is autonomy and all my health strategies are meant to create it. **Figure 47** represents my theory of health in an elementary way. It misses out a lot, and gives

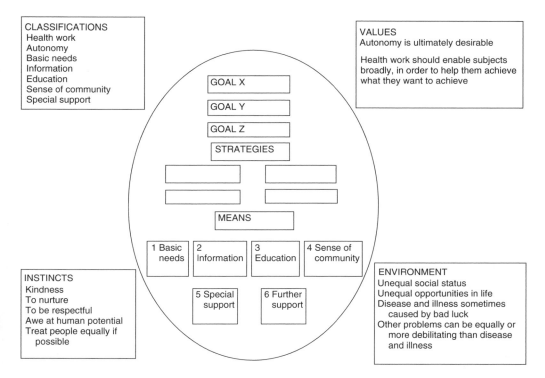

Figure 47 A crude illustration of my foundations understanding of health (the outer rectangles constitute the frame – the rational field is within the ellipse and is created and held together by the frame)

a highly selective interpretation of the picture frame ('environment' especially), but it nevertheless illustrates how my thought and feeling about health creates logical fields of action.

In contrast to my view, medical students are taught that health is the absence of disease (**Figure 48**).

Identical and similar rational fields are regularly created by the different frames shown in **Figures 47** and **48**, giving a false and unfortunate impression of general concord.

Consider a simple example:

> Simon, aged 19, is carried unconscious into an A&E department. His distraught mother says he's swallowed a bottle of paracetamol and left a suicide note.

At this point both the foundations frame and the medical frame will almost certainly create an identical rational field – that in order to work for Simon's health his stomach should be pumped and an antidote to paracetamol administered.

But let events move on:

> Simon recovers. He says he did not want to be saved. He says he is just as depressed as ever. His mother wants the doctors to place him in a hospital for his own protection.

At this point the medical and foundational rational fields are more likely to differ. A doctor using the medical frame, bolstered as it is by its concentration on risk, normality

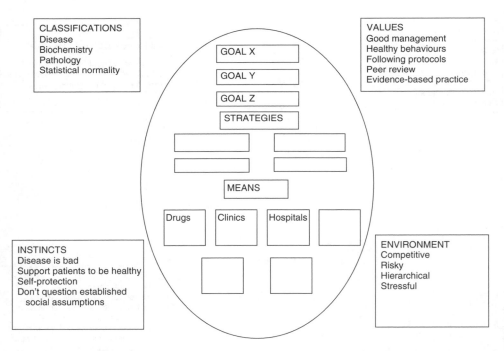

Figure 48 A crude illustration of a generalised medical understanding of health (the outer rectangles constitute the frame – the rational field is within the ellipse and is created and held together by the frame)

and protocol, will probably deem hospitalisation for Simon the best short-term strategy. The foundations frame, on the other hand, might produce a contrasting rational field (dependent partly on a gut decision about which element of the foundations is considered most important). A foundational health worker might take a calculated risk in the interests of Simon's autonomy. She might decide not to further undermine his self-control by hospitalising him, and offer him intensive counselling (away from his mother) in order to build a more robust set of means (Boxes 1–5 in Fig 47) – linking these to short-term goals and strategies Simon can cope with.

Unless the medic and the foundational health worker can see each other's frames (and their own – they must be aware of their own as well) they will remain mystified by how much they disagree.

HOW UNDERSTANDING RATIONALITY LIBERATES US

RATIONALITY IS LOGIC

If you are to be rational it is necessary to have at least one purpose.

In order to pursue your purpose(s) rationally, you should choose the strategy which seems most likely to succeed.

RATIONALITY IS MORE THAN LOGIC

Our purposes do not emanate from logic alone.

Our purposes are created externally to logical reason. They are created (either singly or in some combination) by our biological instincts, by the environments in which we find ourselves, by the language we use to describe the world, and by our values.

In order to understand the nature of rationality it is necessary to see both the logical and the non-logical elements – in other words it is necessary to see both the frame and the picture.

In order to understand yourself it is necessary to understand both the logical and the non-logical elements of your personal rationality – to see what you do and to have at least some sense of why you do it.

In order to understand other people it is necessary to understand both the logical and the non-logical elements of their rationality – to see what they do and to have at least some sense of why they do it.

Even knowing this, it is astonishingly easy to misunderstand ourselves and others. Without knowing this, however, it is INEVITABLE that we will misunderstand ourselves and others.

TO BE TRULY ETHICAL MEANS TO COMMIT KNOWINGLY TO A PARTICULAR SET OF FRAMES

If you just happen to be in a rational field but don't recognise you are in it, then you will either make no moral choices (like a baby) or you will make only those moral choices available to you within that field. For example, you may be a medical doctor routinely working in intensive care, using a set of protocols to decide who to admit. If so you will in a sense be making moral choices, but they will be limited because:

1. You did not design the protocols
2. You have given no thought to entering or creating alternative rational fields in which different choices are possible

Although there may be some morality in choices and actions made within specific rational fields (all social action has ethical content[173]), true morality emanates from decision-makers' AWARENESS of the frames within which they must decide. It is only by transcending the rational field you're in, doing your best to examine the frame which created it, and comparing it with alternative frames and fields, that real moral choice begins.

Three levels of morality (or the importance of moral encounters of the third kind)

It is helpful to distinguish three levels of morality:

1. None
2. Within-field morality
3. Trans-field morality

I believe we should constantly strive for moral encounters of the third kind.

Consider this illustration. If I am a conscripted private in an army, if I can conceive of no other place to be, and if I follow orders whatever they are, then I am exhibiting little and arguably **no moral choice**. If I begin to deliberate about which orders it is ethical to follow then I am becoming morally aware. If I disobey orders I consider immoral then I am exhibiting **within-field morality** (the same applies if I consider orders moral and consequently obey them). If I come to recognise that I inhabit a vast rational field known as 'the army', and if I begin to examine its frame, then I am moving into **trans-field morality**. As I begin to examine the frame's components I enter a condition where I can decide whether to commit to this frame (and its implications) or not. Indeed, once I begin to see a range of rational fields and their frames there is no longer anywhere to hide from morality – I MUST decide which frames to commit to, or I MUST set out to create new rational fields in accord with a frame I have created myself. Once you can see over the walls of specific rational fields your moral life becomes mature and – as a consequence – much, much more difficult.

COMMITMENT

I write in this book (p. 56):

> ...it is possible to see dwarfing as immoral only within a framework of values and reasoning that considers it to be so...WITHIN the foundations theory of health[81] dwarfing is indubitably immoral because according to the foundations theory the central point of working for health is to create autonomy...Yet outside this special framework, dwarfing may or may not be immoral – it all depends on the particular moral framework from which actions are viewed.[74]

I prefer pacifism over aggression, yet if an aggressor has undertaken **trans-field morality** and authentically committed to her preferred rational fields, then she is as moral as I am. This is why it is so desperately important to recognise that:

WORK FOR HEALTH REQUIRES MORAL COMMITMENT

> ... no one is morally obliged to act in any particular way – if you want to behave selfishly no 'moral court' will ever punish you. However, since all social behaviours take place in the moral realm, we continually have a golden opportunity to commit to moral ways of life – if we choose. Those who genuinely wish to work for health must make a knowing commitment to achieving health goals – and this requires commitment to a theory of health. As she commits, the health worker pledges simultaneously to a powerful set of moral obligations – a commitment all the more emphatic because it is voluntary.[77]

Note: the expression 'to behave selfishly' can be taken to mean to act wholly in your own interests in any of the three senses of morality. 'Moral ways of life' can be taken to mean ways of life chosen following **trans-field** reflection.

Ultimately it is COMMITMENT based on **trans-field** reflection that counts, NOT the nature of particular rational fields. Ultimately, rationality is commitment.

References

1. Feyerabend, Paul (1999). *Conquest of Abundance*, Chicago: University of Chicago Press.
2. http://www.sciencesbookreview.com/Conquest_of_Abundance_A_Tale_of_Abstraction_versus_the_Richness_of_Being_0226245349.html *Omar N. Ali*
3. Seedhouse, D.F. (1996). What Good is a Blunt Surgeon? *Health Matters*, Issue **28**, 25.
4. Simon, H.A. (1969). *The Sciences of the Artificial*, Cambridge, MA: MIT Press, pp. 24–5.
5. Ibid., pp. 52–3.
6. Weizenbaum, J. (1984). *Computer Power and Human Reason*, Harmondsworth: Penguin Books, p. 127.
7. Huxley, Aldous (1946). *Science, Liberty, and Peace*, New York: Harper, pp. 35–6.
8. Ibid., pp. 36–7.
9. Rokeach, M. (1973). *The Nature of Human Values*, New York: The Free Press, p. ix.
10. Allport, G.W. (1961). *Pattern and Growth in Personality*, New York: Holt, Rinhart & Winston, p. 454.
11. Rokeach, M. (1973). *The Nature of Human Values*, New York: The Free Press, p. 17.
12. Veatch, Robert M. (1995). Abandoning informed consent. Hastings Center Report; Mar/Apr, **25** Issue 2, p. 5, 8pp.
13. *Star Trek* legend.
14. http://www.marketaz.co.uk/StarTrek/Vulcan/Spock.html
15. http://philosophy.wisc.edu/simplicity/
16. http://www.computing.co.uk/analysis/1143386
17. http://www.cut-the-knot.org/proofs/index.shtml
18. Heudebert, G.R., Van Ruiswyk, J., Hiatt, J. and Schectman, G. (1993). Combination drug therapy for hypercholesterolemia. The trade-off between cost and simplicity. *Arch Intern Med.*, **153**(15): 1828–37.
19. http://www.livingvalues.net/values/simplicity.htm
20. http://www.nwei.org/pages/simplicity.html
21. http://www.naturaltheology.net/Development/Dev02_Model/model04Simplicity.html
22. http://plato.stanford.edu/entries/simplicity/
23. Seedhouse, D.F. (1998). *Ethics: The Heart of Health Care* – QALYs chapter, Chichester: John Wiley.
24. Adapted from: http://www.mindtools.com/pages/article/newTED_04.htm
25. Dr Ray Naden, New Zealand Ministry of Health Consultant, personal communication.
26. Nutt, P.C. (2002). *Why Decisions Fail: Avoiding the Blunders and Traps that Lead to Debacles*, New York: Berrett-Koehler.
27. http://www.princeton.edu/~mdaniels/PD/PD.html
28. http://www.pjhealy.com/coldwar/arms.html
29. Weisbrod, G., Vary, D. and Treyz, G. (2001). *Economic Implications of Road Congestion*, National Cooperative Highway Research Program, Report 463, Washington, DC: National Academy Press.
30. http://www.aibs.org/washington-watch/washington_watch_1995_12.html

31. Kraines, David and Kraines, Vivian (1993). Learning to Cooperate with Pavlov: an Adaptive Strategy for the Iterated Prisoner's Dilemma with Noise, *Theory and Decision*, **35**: 107–50.
32. Carnap, R. (1950). *The Logical Foundations of Probability Theory*, 1962 edn, Chicago: University of Chicago Press.
33. Simon, H.A. et al. (1986). *Research Briefings 1986: Report of the Research Briefing Panel on Decision Making and Problem Solving*, National Academy of Sciences, Washington, DC: National Academy Press.
34. http://www2.sjsu.edu/faculty/watkins/prospect.htm
35. Bentham, J. (1789). Introduction to the Principles of Morals and Legislation, Chapter 4.
36. Mautner, Thomas (ed.) (1996). *A Dictionary of Philosophy* (a revised and corrected version of the hardback edition, Oxford: Blackwell). London: Penguin, 1997, xix + 482 pp. Re-impressions with minor changes 1998, 1999, 2000, 2002.
37. http://www.utilitarian.org/maths.html
38. http://www.mind.ilstu.edu/misc/morality/zydek/design.html
39. *Journal of the American Medical Association* (1997), **277**: 519–20.
40. http://www.nih.gov/
41. http://consensus.nih.gov/cons/103/103_intro.htm
42. http://www.acsh.org/healthissues/newsID.765/healthissue_detail.asp
43. Final mammography recommendation? *Journal of the American Medical Association* (1997), **277**: 1181.
44. Money, G., Jan, S. and Wiseman, V. (1995). Examining preferences for allocating health care gains, *Health Care Analysis*, **3**(3), 261–5.
45. Williams, A. (1995). Health economics and health care priorities, *Health Care Analysis*, **3**(3), 221–34.
46. Farrar, S., Donaldson, D., Macphee, S., Walker, A. and Mapp, T. (1997). Riposte. Creativity and sacrifice: two sides of the coin. A reply to David Seedhouse, *Health Care Analysis*, **5**(4), 306–9.
47. Donaldson, C., Farrar, S., Walker, A., Mapp, T. and Macphee, S. (1997). Assessing community values in health care: is the 'willingness to pay' method feasible? *Health Care Analysis*, **5**(1), 7–29.
48. Russell, Bertrand (1947). *History of Western Philosophy and Its Connection with Political and Social Circumstances from the Earliest Times to the Present Day*, London: George Allen & Unwin.
49. http://www.college.columbia.edu/core/lectures/fall1999/index.php
50. Lee, D. (1955). *Plato: The Republic*, translated with an introduction by Desmond Lee. Harmondsworth: Penguin Books.
51. Cottingham, J., Stoothoff, R. and Murdoch, D. (1984). *The Philosophical Writings of Descartes*. Cambridge: Cambridge University Press.
52. Popper, K. (1977). *The Open Society and Its Enemies*, Vol. 2, London: Routledge & Kegan Paul, p. 234.
53. Weizenbaum, J. (1984). *Computer Power and Human Reason: From Judgement to Calculation*, London: Pelican Books, pp. 215–16.
54. Damasio, A. (1994). *Descartes' Error*, New York: Grosset/Putnam.
55. Ibid., p. 10.
56. Ibid., p. 134.
57. Ibid., p. 200.
58. Ibid., p. 173.
59. Kelley, L. Ross. http://www.friesian.com/founda-1.htm
60. Hume, D. (1740). *A Treatise of Human Nature*, 1978 edn, Bk. II, Part III, Oxford University Press, p. 156.
61. Dowie, J. http://www.collegiumramazzini.org/links/DOWIE.PDF
62. Seedhouse, D.F. (2003). War is for reptiles, *Health Matters*, **51**: 25.
63. Seedhouse, D.F. (2003). *Health Promotion: Philosophy, Prejudice and Practice*, 2nd edn, Chichester: John Wiley.
64. American Psychiatric Association (2000). *Diagnostic and Statistical Manual of Mental Disorders*, 4th edn (DSM IV), Washington, DC: American Psychiatric Press.
65. DSM IV, p. 90.
66. Szasz, T. (1974). *The Myth of Mental Illness*, New York: Harper & Row.
67. DSM IV, p. xxiii.
68. DSM IV, pp. 83–4.
69. Wittgenstein, L. (1958). *Philosophical Investigations*, Oxford, Basil Blackwell & Mott.
70. Hollis, M. and Lukes, S. (1982). *Rationality and Relativism*, Oxford: Basil Blackwell, p. 7.

71. Ibid., p. 9.
72. Ibid., p. 10.
73. *Stanford Encyclopaedia of Philosophy*, http://plato.stanford.edu/entries/moral-relativism/
74. Woodbridge, K. and Fulford, K.W.M. (2004). *Whose Values? A workbook for values-based practice in mental health care*, The Sainsbury Centre for Mental Health.
75. http://www.september11news.com/
76. http://newswww.bbc.net.uk/1/hi/world/europe/3741434.stm
77. Seedhouse, D.F. (1998). *Ethics: The Heart of Health Care*, 2nd edn, Chichester: John Wiley.
78. Ibid., pp. 87–8.
79. Ibid., p. 98.
80. Ibid., pp. 99–101.
81. Seedhouse, D.F. (2001). *Health: The Foundations for Achievement*, 2nd edn, Chichester: John Wiley.
82. American Cancer Society (2001). Cancer facts and figures. Available at: http://www.cancer.org/downloads/STT/F&F2001.pdf.
83. Gail, M., Brinton, L.A., Byar, D.P. et al. (1989). Projecting individualized probabilities of developing breast cancer for white females who are being examined annually. *J. Natl. Cancer Inst.*, **81**: 1879–86.
84. Colditz, G.A., Willett, W.C., Hunter, D.J. et al. (1993). Family history, age, and risk of breast cancer. Prospective data from the Nurses' Health Study [published erratum appears in *JAMA*, 1993; **270**(13): 1548], *JAMA*, **270**(3): 338–43.
85. Seidman, H., Stellman, S.D. and Mushinski, M.H. (1982). A different perspective on breast cancer risk factors: some implications of the nonattributable risk. *Cancer*, **32**: 301–12.
86. Strax, P. (1987). Mass screening of asymptomatic women. In: Ariel, I.M. and Cleary, J. (eds), *Breast Cancer: Diagnosis and Treatment*, New York: McGraw-Hill, pp. 145–51.
87. http://www.ahrq.gov/clinic/3rduspstf/breastcancer/bcscrnsum1.htm
88. Ereshefsky, M. (ed.) (1992). *The Units of Evolution: Essays on the Nature of the Species*, Cambridge, MA: MIT Press.
89. Blakely, R. (1996). *Potential Theory in Gravity and Magnetic Applications*, Cambridge: Cambridge University Press.
90. Guterson, D. (1993). *Family Matters: Why Homeschooling Makes Sense*, New York: Harcourt Brace, Harvest edn, p. 177.
91. Cohen, P. (2000). Is the addiction doctor the voodoo priest of the Western man? Extended version of an article in *Addiction Research*, special issue, **8**, 6. See: wysiwyg://www.cedro-uva.org/lib/cohen.addiction.html
92. http://www.ihs.ox.ac.uk/ebh/ebh1b.html Institute of Health Sciences, University of Oxford.
93. Seedhouse, D.F. (2002). Total Health Promotion: Mental Health, Rational Field and the Quest for Autonomy, Chichester: John Wiley.
94. Jarvie, I.C. (1970). Explaining Cargo Cults, in *Rationality*, ed. Bryan R. Wilson, Oxford: Basil Blackwell.
95. Jarvie, I.C. and Agassi, J. (1970). The Problem of the Rationality of Magic, in ibid.
96. Kekes, I. (1976). *A Justification of Rationality*, Albany, NY: State University of New York Press.
97. Seedhouse, D.F. (1984). *Rationality*, PhD Thesis, Manchester University (unpublished).
98. Camazine, S. (1992). *Self-organisation in Biological Systems*, Princeton, NJ: Princeton University Press.
99. Seedhouse, D.F. (2003). *Health Promotion: Philosophy, Prejudice and Practice*, 2nd edn, Chichester: John Wiley.
100. Collins, Patricia Hill (1990). *Black Feminist Thought: Knowledge, Consciousness, and the Politics of Empowerment*. New York: Routledge.
101. http://www.webster-dictionary.org/definition/Discourse
102. http://www.retroweb.com/prisoner.html
103. Orwell, G. (2002). *1984*, Harmondsworth: Penguin Books.
104. http://www.online-literature.com/orwell/1984/48
105. Koestler, A. (1979). *Janus: A Summing Up*, London: Pan Books.
106. Wilson, C. (1979). *The Occult*, London: Granada Publishing.
107. http://members.aol.com/mcnelis/Medsci/cathsci.html
108. http://www.guardian.co.uk/gender/story/0,11812,1356386,00.html
109. Leibrich, J. (ed.) (1999). *A Gift of Stories*, University of Otago Press.
110. Breggin, P.R. (1994). *Toxic Psychiatry*, New York: St. Martins Press.

111. http://www.ace.ac.nz/doclibrary/pdf/postgraduate/staff/erata/MaoriLanguageRevivalNZ Education.pdf
112. Smith, L.T. (1994). Kaupapa Maori Research, unpublished paper, Auckland University, pp. 1–2.
113. http://www.moh.govt.nz/moh.nsf/0/ffc06a2c2009deeecc256b9400787b61?OpenDocument
114. Maui Hudson (2004). Unpublished paper, Auckland University of Technology.
115. http://www.hartford-hwp.com/archives/28/063.html
116. http://www.kcl.ac.uk/depsta/ccm/CCM_mentalhealth.html
117. http://www.fpanet.org/journal/articles/1999_Issues/jfp0399-art12.cfm (*Journal of Financial Planning*).
118. **Institute for International Relations Conference, Ottawa, 3–5 October 2000**, Governance and Accountability in the Public Sector – Balancing Social, Political and Business Pressures during Times of Change, Janice Cochrane, Deputy Minister of Citizenship and Immigration, Co-Champion of Values and Ethics in the Public Service.) See: http://www.hrma-agrh.gc.ca/veo-bve/speeches/intlrelationconf_e.asp
119. http://corporate.smartpros.com/education/workingvalues/vbe.html
120. Downie, R.S., Fyfe, C. and Tannahill, A. (1990). *Health Promotion: Models and Values*, Oxford University Press, Oxford.
121. Little, J.M. (2002), *Medical Journal of Australia*, **177**(6): 319–21.
122. Bernstein, P. (1998). *Against the Gods: The remarkable story of risk* (Vols 92–95). New York: John Wiley.
123. http://www.pollingreport.com/
124. http://www.ontargetresearch.com/
125. Drummond, M.F., O'Brien, B.J., Stoddart, G.L. and Torrence, G.W. (1997). *Methods for the Economic Evaluation of Health Care Programmes*, 2nd edn., Oxford University Press, New York.
126. http://www.deliberative-mapping.org/
127. http://www.guidetopsychology.com/testing.htm
128. http://82.219.38.131/ukcp.org.uk/home.asp
129. Arrigo, B. (2000). *Introduction to Forensic Psychology: Issues and Controversies in Crime and Justice*. New York: Academic Press.
130. Fenton S. Martin (c 1999). *CQ's Resource Guide to Modern Elections: an Annotated Bibliography, 1960–1996*, Washington, DC: CQ Press.
131. Developing a Value-Based Decision-Making Model for Inquiring Organizations, Dianne Hall, Auburn University, Yi Guo, Texas A&M University, Robert A. Davis, Southwest Texas State University. Abstract: http://csdl.computer.org/comp/proceedings/hicss/2003/1874/04/187440111aabs.htm Full paper: http://csdl.computer.org/comp/proceedings/hicss/2003/1874/04/187440111a.pdf
132. http://eetd.lbl.gov/btp/papers/45548.pdf
133. http://www.uacil.com/actionpoint.html, http://www.uacil.com/pressreleases.html
134. http://www.connects.org.uk/conferences/conference_papers.asp?codeItemID=12&profile Code=00020001
135. The principles and practice of Values-Based Medicine are described in Fulford, K.W.M. (forthcoming) *Values-Based Medicine: Effective Healthcare Decision-Making in the Context of Value Diversity*, Cambridge: Cambridge University Press.
136. http://hsc.unm.edu/~hsethics/pubbennett.htm
137. Seedhouse, D.F. (2000). *Practical Nursing Philosophy: The Universal Ethical Code*, Chichester: John Wiley.
138. Annas, J. (2003). Virtue Ethics and Social Psychology, *A Priori*, Vol. 2, pp. 20–34.
139. http://www.umich.edu/~newsinfo/MT/01/Fal01/mt6f01.html
140. http://www.edsource.org/pub_edfct_polls.cfm
141. Brannigan, M. (1993). Oregon's Experiment, *Health Care Analysis*, **1**:1: 15–32.
142. http://www.apma.org/code.htm, http://www.med.nyu.edu/compliance/ethical.html
143. http://www.adolescenthealth.org/researchethics.htm
144. Kent, G. (1997). The views of members of Local Research Ethics Committees, researchers and members of the public towards the roles and functions of LRECs, *Journal of Medical Ethics*, **23**: 186–90.
145. James, T. and Platzer, H. (1999). Ethical considerations in qualitative research with vulnerable groups: exploring lesbians' and gay men's experiences of health care – a personal perspective', *Nursing Ethics*, **6**, 1: 73–81.

146. Seedhouse, D.F. and Gallagher, A. (2002). Undignifying Institutions, *Journal of Medical Ethics*, **28**: 368–72.
147. http://www.whale.to/v/menin5.html
148. Beauchamp, T.L. and Childress, J.F. (2001). *Principles of Biomedical Ethics*, 5th edn, Oxford: Oxford University Press.
149. http://news.bbc.co.uk/1/hi/health/background_briefings/the_bristol_heart_babies/297182.stm
150. www.westerncity.com Contact: Patty Chazen pchazen@cacities.org
151. http://www.magistrates-assoc-kent.fsnet.co.uk/Sentencing.htm
152. http://www.idmu.co.uk/roulette.htm
153. http://lifeissues.net/writers/fin/fin_01aborcloneevasions.html
154. *Judge Questions Long Sentence in Drug Case, The New York Times*, 17 November 2004.
155. Shamberg, Johnson and Bergman, A. (1996). *Quarterly Newsletter*, **4**, No. 3 (Summer) p. 7.
156. http://www.cnn.com/2004/WORLD/meast/01/25/sprj.nirq.kay/
157. Deci, E.L. and Ryan, R.M. (1985). *Intrinsic Motivation and Self-determination in Human Behavior*. New York: Plenum.
158. Pelletier, L.G., Tuson, K.M. and Haddad, N.K. (1997). Client Motivation for Therapy Scale: A measure of intrinsic motivation, extrinsic motivation and amotivation for therapy. *Journal of Personality Assessment*, **68**: 414–35.
159. Ryan, R.M. and Connell, J.P. (1989). Perceived locus of causality and internalization: Examining reasons for acting in two domains. *Journal of Personality and Social Psychology*, **57**: 749–61.
160. Ryan, R.M., Plant, R.W. and O'Malley, S. (1995). Initial motivations for alcohol treatment: Relations with patient characteristics, treatment involvement and dropout. *Addictive Behaviors*, **20**: 279–97.
161. Williams, G.C., Cox, E.M., Kouides, R. and Deci, E.L. (1999). Presenting the facts about smoking to adolescents: The effects of an autonomy supportive style. *Archives of Pediatrics and Adolescent Medicine*, **153**: 959–64.
162. Williams, G.C., Deci, E.L. and Ryan, R.M. (1998). Building Health-Care Partnerships by Supporting Autonomy: Promoting Maintained Behavior Change and Positive Health Outcomes. In A.L. Suchman, P. Hinton-Walker & R. Botelho (eds), *Partnerships in Healthcare: Transforming Relational Process*, Rochester, NY: University of Rochester Press, pp. 67–87.
163. Williams, G.C., Freedman, Z.R. and Deci, E.L. (1998). Supporting autonomy to motivate glucose control in patients with diabetes. *Diabetes Care*, **21**: 1644–51.
164. Williams, G.C., Grow, V.M., Freedman, Z., Ryan, R.M. and Deci, E.L. (1996). Motivational predictors of weight loss and weight-loss maintenance. *Journal of Personality and Social Psychology*, **70**, 115–26.
165. Williams, G.C., Rodin, G.C., Ryan, R.M., Grolnick, W.S. and Deci, E.L. (1998). Autonomous regulation and long-term medication adherence in adult outpatients. *Health Psychology*, **17**: 269–76.
166. Zeldman, A., Ryan, R.M. and Fiscella, K. (1999). Attitudes, beliefs and motives in addiction recovery. Unpublished manuscript, University of Rochester.
167. *Star Trek* (original series, first broadcast 16 Nov 1967): Journey To Babel.
168. Seedhouse, D.F. (1984). *Rationality*, PhD Thesis, Manchester University (unpublished), pp. ii–iii.
169. http://dictionary.reference.com/search?q=rationality
170. http://dictionary.cambridge.org/define.asp?key=65573&dict=CALD
171. Seedhouse, D.F. (2001). *Health: The Foundations for Achievement*, 2nd edn, Chichester: John Wiley, pp. 30–1.
172. Seedhouse, D.F. (1984). *Rationality*, PhD Thesis. Manchester University (unpublished), pp. 112–13.
173. Seedhouse, D.F. (1998). *Ethics: The Heart of Health Care*, 2nd edn, Chichester: John Wiley, pp. 7–8.

Index

Page numbers in *italic* indicate figures.

The Seedhouse Bookshelf Collection

Invaluable resources for medical, nursing and other health professionals and students.

Health Promotion
Philosophy, Prejudice and Practice
Second Edition
This book examines why, in practice, the delivery of health promotion information is ambiguous and contradictory. The new edition includes: *New chapters and teaching exercises *Incorporates and updates the guide for teachers and lecturers *A new topical case study.
0-470-84732-8 November 2003 320pp Hbk
0-470-84733-6 November 2003 320pp Pbk

Total Health Promotion
Mental Health, Rational Fields and the Quest for Autonomy
"...you will find this book both accessible and thought provoking. Put Total Health Promotion high on your books to read – you won't be disappointed."
JOURNAL OF THE ROYAL SOCIETY FOR THE PROMOTION OF HEALTH, JUNE 2003
In this unique and remarkable book Seedhouse has developed an exciting and potentially revolutionary health promotion tool – the rational field. Simple to use rational fields enable health promoters to plan and act in total honesty, using whatever methods are best suited to their quest to create autonomy.
0-471-49013-X August 2002 170pp Pbk

Health
The Foundations for Achievement
Second Edition
"...You will find it not only intellectually exciting but also highly thought-provoking..."
JOURNAL OF THE ROYAL SOCIETY FOR THE PROMOTION OF HEALTH, SEPTEMBER 2002
This inspirational book poses two fundamental questions – "What is health?" and "How can more health be achieved?" – and answers them at a depth unmatched by any other text in this field.
0-471-49011-3 May 2001 160pp Pbk

Practical Nursing Philosophy
The Universal Ethical Code
"To me, a non-nurse, this is an excellent, clear book..."
NURSING ETHICS, VOL 8/3, 2001
A precise yet compassionate framework that enables nurses to reflect deeply about the importance of their work, and can support them as they strive to make ethically sound decisions.
0-471-49012-1 September 2000 234pp Pbk

Ethics
The Heart of Health Care
Second Edition
A classic ethics text in medical, health and nursing studies – is recommended around the globe for its straightforward introduction to ethical analysis.
0-471-97592-3 March 1998 250pp Pbk

Also of interest:

Health: The Foundations of Achievement, D.F. Seedhouse, 1986
Changing Ideas in Health Care, Eds D.F. Seedhouse and A. Cribb, 1989
Liberating Medicine, D.F. Seedhouse, 1991
Practical Medical Ethics, D.F. Seedhouse and L. Lovett, 1992
Reforming Health Care: The Philosophy and Practice of International Health Reform, Ed D.F. Seedhouse, 1995
Fortress NHS: A Philosophical Review of the National Health Service, D.F. Seedhouse, 1994